DEBRA'S GIFTS

A story of love. The beginning and end of life.

by Lorraine Paul Noznisky

ISBN

978-1-4602-1808-2 (Hardcover)
978-1-4602-1809-9 (Paperback)
978-1-4602-1810-5 (eBook)

Photographer: Donna Lafornia

Produced by:

FriesenPress

Suite 300 – 852 Fort Street
Victoria, BC, Canada V8W 1H8

www.friesenpress.com

Distributed to the trade by The Ingram Book Company

Table of Contents

DEDICATION

To those who love, who are loved, and who know why.

A portion of the proceeds of this book will be donated in Debra's name to the following:

Mercy Flight Western New York *(www.mercyflightwny.com)*

May she soar through the sky and through the clouds and see the children and people that she will help. Thank you!

CCS Foundation, Inc., Williamsville, NY

—

FOREWORD

Mother's Statement:

This book is our experience in the walk of cancer. It began the first day my daughter, Debra, was diagnosed. Never did I think that my diary would serve any purpose other than to try to understand the mystery and confusions, lack of information, or misinformation during her treatments, and our hopes, disappointments, and the roller-coaster of emotions. The confusing medications — so foreign as neither Debra or I had to take during our lives. We have never been able to verify her treatments, as after numerous requests, we were not given Debra's medical records.

My daughter was not being tested every year. I look back and wonder how I missed this. Am I left with the guilt that I never asked her? Could anybody else have loved her enough to make her go to a doctor? However, she was strong-willed.

I feel we could have been more proactive in her treatment, researched other methods of treatment, asked about the treatments, or why subject her to this poison in the first place if the end result would have been the same. Were we told the truth? We will forever have these doubts. We never realized that the word "Institute" means a teaching hospital. Oh, my, God! Then the maze of unfamiliar procedures, medications, and phrases that the medical field toss out and leave in the air. Warning: This book contains graphic descriptions.

My sincere prayer is that the information will help families receiving this frightening news. I implore young women to keep annual gynecological tests — PLEASE! Don't ever put yourself or your loved ones through this experience. Their inner circle can influence this action. Stop smoking! Get tested annually!

Also, please do the Internet research. These medical references should be used as a base to discuss with your physician. I am not, nor is the source of my research, responsible for the content of the information. That responsibility falls to you.

And as you hold this book in your hands and close your eyes at its conclusion, raise a prayer for my daughter, Debra. She was a joy — a gift.

2/19/12

THE NEWS!

"NO! NO! NO! PLEASE, GOD, NO!" I screamed as I dropped the speaker phone back in the cradle. I was sobbing; I fell to my knees by the side of the bed. My husband, Jerr, had tears, too. He just stroked my hair. I couldn't believe what we had just been told by the doctor. Why? After all this time, why?

A million thoughts and memories raced through my head. The doctors had always said that everything was going fine, but "Let's have more treatments, more tests, more medications, more hospitalizations, but everything will be fine." Now I hated all of them. I was pounding my fists into the bedspread, saying how much I hated the doctors and the hospitals and the phony people connected with them. I said the three swear words I knew, surprising Jerr who had never heard such language from me. Jerr said, "Sweetheart, we can't let this destroy us. We have to be loving and strong like we've always been. We have to show Debbie our love like we've always done."

I thought what do we do? We have to leave Florida now! How do we get back to her this instant? How long will it take? How can I tell her? Who do we talk to — a multitude of questions? I wrapped my arms around my stomach, and I could feel my daughter, Debra. I could feel her as I did when I first held her in my arms.

PROLOGUE
1959 - 1960
THE BEGINNING OF LOVE

Mother's memory - 6/28

What a gift I received when the nurses put a tiny bundle of baby girl in my arms. I felt terrified. I felt excited. She was so tiny. All I could see in that pink blanket was a cap of light brown/blonde hair and her eyelashes, long and curly down on her soft cheeks brushing luminous, silky skin. Then she opened her hazel eyes, and I knew, I knew right then she smiled at me and held on to my finger. That was it — true love. She was all mine and I christened her Debra Lynn, my daughter.

11/26 - Then seventeen months later, I received the gift of another tiny girl born with dark hair, dark eyelashes and mysterious eyes. We named her Donna Marie. She resembled her father — my husband, who I met when he attended dental college. Our marriage lasted nineteen years. For thirty years, I had never wanted to put a Mrs. in front of my name until I met the man who gently changed the 3rd phase of my life.

> *The moment a child is born,*
> *the mother is also born.*
> *She never existed before.*
> *The woman existed but the mother, never.*

A mother is something absolutely new.

Rajneesh

The two girls changed my life forever. My life was now not about me but about them. I prayed that I would be worthy of such gifts. As a child, Debra was precocious, making statements like what she wanted to do, where to go or what to eat, and Donna would say, "Me, too." Donna was known as "me, too." Her grandfather would say, "Bring the girls over — you know, Debra and "me, too". In photos of the two of them all dressed in their matching Easter finery and bonnets, or Christmas with Santa, or whatever holiday it was, Debra was holding baby Donna, people would think, Donna was Debra's doll. They were always together — right from the beginning.

But on that June 28, I thought about what in the world was I going to do with this gift. My mind traveled back to another beginning......

Debra's father had disappeared after our 3-day marriage one year before. We had known each other for two and a half years. Over the years, I had spoken to his family only a couple of times as he was obligated to call home every Friday. I never got the sense that they were a close loving family; he would reach for the phone, take a breath, and say "Well, here goes." Their conversations lasted only a few minutes — "How are you, mother? How is father? What news is there? Talk to you next week. Bye." Where were the "I love you" statements?

We were married at Los Angeles City Hall with my cousin and her husband as witnesses and the four of us spent the weekend together sightseeing. Two days after he returned to the Marine base, the calls stopped. After several weeks his best friend called me to inform me that the weekend after our wedding, my husband's parents had flown in from Texas and had somehow arranged to have him transferred to Virginia where he entered OCS and that "they" were annulling the marriage. He was 24 years old! What must they have told him to influence him not to even try to contact me in any way? What control did they have? Well, what a gift he missed.

2009

THE DIAGNOSIS

4/9/09 to 4/17/09, Thurs. to Thurs. — Florida

What a gift of this time! For years, my husband, Jerry, (Jerr), and I had anticipated a visit from a member of our family, and finally it was Debra and her son, Jeremy, who came to spend Jeremy's spring break with us. Jerr and I had given them the Christmas gift of Jet Blue flights from a cold, freezing Buffalo, New York to sunny Ft. Lauderdale, Florida. It was to be their first flight together. Debra and Jeremy were so close. They loved each other so much, and it was a joy to see them together, talking, sharing, asking, telling, laughing. They were so excited. Debra later told us that right after the plane's take-off and few hard bumps, Jeremy had asked her, "Mom, what if the plane crashes?" She held his hand and said "Well, then we'll be together forever." 🏝️ 🏝️

Jerr and I were happy to have them with us. I made up a sign — "DEBRA & JEREMY" — like the ones the limousine drivers have at the arrivals area of airports. We arrived at the airport hours early — we didn't want to miss them. Finally, we could see them walking down the long hallway in the arrivals area. We pretended to look over their heads and behind them, as if we didn't see them. When they spotted us, there were smiles and then laughter about the sign, hugs, and then more smiles and finally getting to the luggage kiosk. When we walked out into the lovely bright sunshine, Debra and Jeremy both looked up to the sky so the warm sun was on their throats, and they were amazed at the swaying palm trees. They looked at each other and were still smiling. Jeremy is a quiet person but he doesn't miss anything. He was observing everything around him.

4/9/09, Thurs. —

Jeremy asked if we could stop at one of his favorite places for breakfast, McDonald's. At home, we spent the afternoon at the pool, which overlooks the Intracoastal Waterway, where they both fell asleep on the lounges. We had a light lunch under the canopy. After dinner, we sat talking and laughing. An early night as everyone agreed we were all tired. "Good night, Mom and Jerr. We love you." "*We love you, too.*"

4/10/09, Fri. **— Easter Weekend**

Because of the holiday, we hadn't planned anything significant. We spent more time at the pool just lounging out there, taking naps; they loved it. I prepared another picnic lunch, then back to the pool and the lounges. Jerr and I remained under the canopy — I was reading, and he had his earphones listening to his favorite Cuban radio stations. I kept watching Debra and Jeremy so they wouldn't get sunburned as they are both light-skinned.

Dinner tonight was with my best friend, Terri, and Mark, at the ARK Hollywood (Asian). Lots of laughs and good food!

4/11/09, Sat. —

Debra and I shopped for Jeremy's surprise Easter basket items. Jerr and I had shopped earlier in the week for him and had not only special candies but other surprises. We had a small dinner at home.

4/12/09, Sun. — EASTER SUNDAY.

Jeremy awoke to his surprise Easter basket! He came out of the bedroom with a smile on his face and said, "Thank you!" I love when Jeremy smiles; he has one of those beaming smiles. We all had special Easter cards at our breakfast table setting. I served toasted challah bread, which Jerr had introduced to Jeremy and Debra; they loved it. I attended Mass at St. Matthew Church.

Another pool day and then we prepared for dinner at China Buffet with our delightful 95-year old friend, Alice. During dinner, Jeremy laughed when Jerr put his crab claws near Alice's cheek like it was going to pinch her. She jumped, then started laughing, and picked up her crab legs and went after Jerr, and they started a "sword" fight! We were all laughing. ⚔ ⚔ (*Months later, Debra said Jeremy never forgot that dinner and the crab claws. We had cancelled dinner at Joseph's because the kids wanted a casual dinner, and Debra wanted that instead of a traditional Easter dinner at home. We certainly didn't mind.*)

Much later that evening, we were sitting in the bedroom and telling stories and reminiscing. "Mom, do you know what Jeremy remembers when he was a little boy? The "invisible ball!" And we started laughing.

(*When Jeremy was a little boy, Jerr played a game called the "invisible ball". Jerr would tell Jeremy to throw him a "ball", and Jerr would catch it in the brown sandwich bag. Jeremy didn't want to do it until we showed him how. I tossed the "ball" to Jerr and he would catch it in the bag. Jeremy looked in the bag and .....no ball. Now he was fascinated and started throwing the "ball" to Jerr and no matter how high or fast or loopy he would throw the ball, Jerry would catch it in the bag. Jeremy kept looking in the bag and.....no ball. Finally, Jerr showed Jeremy the trick. When he held the bag and the ball is tossed, you snap your fingers and it sounds like a ball dropped into the bag!*)

And laughing from the living room, Jerr called out, "What about the magic garage door opener?" We said, "Oh yes, oh yes."

Jerry would keep the garage door opener in his pocket and press it so the door would open. Jeremy kept looking and trying to figure out how he could sit in the car yet open the door without using his hands. Eventually, Jerr showed Jeremy the garage door opener and after the dozens of questions about how it worked, Jeremy would spend minutes opening and closing the door repeatedly — and I looked at Jerr and said, "Jerrrrrrryyyyyyyy!"

Then the "hold your head" game when we passed under a railroad bridge and a train was passing overhead. At every railroad bridge, Jeremy would put his hands on his head and say "Hold your head!"

Lots of laughs and finally after midnight, we all settled down. I could hear Debra and Jeremy quietly talking and giggles.

4/13/09, Mon. —

At the Broadwalk at the beautiful Hollywood Beach, Jerr took Jeremy to the edge of the beach for his first dip in the Atlantic Ocean. We walked for hours, stopping for lunch, more walking, pedaling the tricycles, and after an afternoon rest and ice cream — we returned home tired but so happy. That evening after dinner, Debra and Jeremy went swimming, and we sat at under the canopy or around the pool for hours watching the yachts go by, so close you could almost touch them. They were ablaze with lights and music. We watched the Intracoastal bridge open up for them. We saw all the city lights and watched the stars come out. There was a lovely warm breeze and it was delightfully quiet. Again, to bed after midnight.

4/14/09, Tues. —

Debra stopped at the pharmacy for a sunscreen with 50 SPF for Jeremy as she felt the tube we had on hand didn't have a high enough SPF. He was getting red in spite of the sunscreen she applied and with Jeremy's fair skin, Debra was concerned that he not sun burn. (Mom, do you remember when I got sunburned as a kid and had big blisters on my shoulders?)

(Yes, sweetheart, that was before all the warnings regarding the sun, and sun screens, and SPFs. You, Donna and your friends were jumping in and out of our pool and you got sunburned. You had such huge blisters on your shoulders. It was terrible. I couldn't touch you or apply medication or spray; you barely could wear any clothes or Pjs, it was so painful. I was reading on the patio and watching you girls and all your friends. Later, I cried that I even though I had sprayed sunscreen, I hadn't thought of reapplying it. I even sprayed the other girls whose mothers had sent them without sunscreen. But your light skin made you burn the worse.)

At last, we were on our way to Ft. Lauderdale for the famous Jungle Queen cruise with a stop on their island where we had a fast bite for lunch. The cruise took us past the millionaires' houses and finally a return to Ft. Lauderdale for dinner. A very relaxing day.

4/15/09, Wed. —

Following lunch at the Cheesecake Factory, we took a walking tour of the 5-mile long Aventura Mall, eventually rode the trolley from one end of the Mall to another just so we could see all the stores. We did some shopping where Jeremy bought a bronze watch. Later in the afternoon, we stopped for a rest and a hot chocolate at a kiosk.

After a two hour rest, we drove to the Hard Rock Café, where there, too, we walked from one end to the other, inside and outside past the beach, under the grotto and waterfalls, over the bridges, then to the other end where the shops and lake with the colored fountains were programmed to music — it was beautiful. Jeremy bought his souvenir t-shirt and we gifted one for Debra, a black one with the Hard Rock Hollywood words in silver glitter. It became her favorite t-shirt and she loved it and wore it often.

Inside the Hard Rock, one incident was when for a moment,

Jeremy took a couple of steps off the tiled area onto the carpeted casino area to better see the slot machines we were playing. Security came up to him and quietly told him he had to stay in the tiled area because he was a minor. He was not happy! He's tall for his age, but apparently, he was "spotted."

Later that evening, we again went to our pool. Returning home at 10:00 p.m., Debra was not feeling well and had pain in the middle of her back. I called a friend/neighbor, another Debbie, a massage therapist, who gave Debra a 30-minute massage. Debra said she felt super! "Whew, what a relief. Thank you!" Jeremy had spent an evening with Debbie's son where they played video games, and Jeremy said he won.

(I was concerned about Debra's back pain, remembering that in December of 2005 at Debra's place of employment on Grand Island, an apartment complex where she also resided, she was driving from one building to another when she became a victim of a car accident. It was the first ice storm of the season; the roads on the property hadn't been sanded yet. Debra, stopped at the stop sign, saw another resident coming around the curve too fast and swerving and skidding. She remained at the stop sign but he hit her on the driver's side. Since that accident, she had been treated for the injury to her neck and lower back and had finally recovered. Occasional flair-ups necessitated her to have chiropractic treatments. She loved her job but eventually lost it, her apartment, her car and any benefits she had! New York State is a No-Fault state and each person in an accident is responsible to pay their own costs through their individual insurers. The man who hit Debra had no insurance. I wonder if people like this realize that by being irresponsible in their own lives, how they affect the life of others?)

4/16/09, Thurs. — En route to airport

Up at 5:00 a.m., stopped at McDonald's for breakfast sandwiches. At the airport, we hugged and said "We love you" and goodbye to our kids. Sadly, we watched them enter the Security line and then turn and give us a final wave until we couldn't see them any more — not with the tears in my eyes. We remained at the airport until the monitor indicated that the flight had departed. Slowly, we walked away. I cried at the emptiness of our condo.

4/17/09, Fri. — Debra's call

They had returned home with no problems, but they were tired. Jeremy spent the weekend with Debra before he had to return to school. She wasn't feeling well again and was lying down.

"I love you two." *"We love you, too, Debra."*

4/18/09, Sat. — Debra's call

She and Jeremy had talked all the way back on their flight about their trip to Florida. They loved it, had fun, were remembering everything we had done! "Thank you and Jerr again, Mom. You made it so special for us. Jeremy is already talking about next year or this summer or anytime! He was asking when can we come back." ⚓ ⚓

4/21/09, Tues. Call to Debra

There was no answer. I laughingly left a message — "Debra, where in the world are you? Are you flying back to Florida?!

She called later in the evening and said she had not been feeling well and had slept all weekend.

4/26/09, Sun. — Debra's call

She was crying; she had been sick in bed since her return from Florida. "I didn't want to tell you, Mom, because I didn't want to worry you, especially after all the fun we had." When she described her symptoms — cramps and bloody discharge and diarrhea, I told her to go to the hospital immediately. I didn't know what was wrong but knew she needed medical attention.

In Niagara Falls Memorial Medical Hospital (NFMMH). Debra was in the emergency room (E/R) for 12 hours, and then was admitted because of her test results. Her red blood cells* were sky high; the white ones* were very low. She was told there was a blood infection somewhere or she had caught a virus. Her stool analysis indicated she was bleeding from somewhere as there was blood present, and she was dehydrated. She was started on a saline IV, given a CT scan*, and lots of blood tests. They started her on antibiotics and Lortab*. The next day, she was informed her ascending colon* was irritated from the diarrhea.

Debra remembered that she and Jeremy had eaten a sandwich prepared at a kiosk at the airport in New York in between their plane change, and it was right after that when she became sick to her stomach. "Was it spoiled, Mom, or did someone with an infection prepare it? Is that why I have a virus?"

5/1/09, Fri. @ NFMMH —

Debra may be discharged; doctors had ordered many tests. Nurses woke her up at 5:30 a.m. for blood work and informed her she was going for an ultrasound*. She was there for 1-1/2 hours, and then the test took another 1-1/2 hours to set up. The machine took pictures of her gallbladder*, and then dye was injected, I guess to see if her gallbladder was functioning properly. Other tests done were on her kidneys and liver. Because she had a stomach virus, the acids started attacking it, and by doing so, it ate a hole in her stomach. They said the "peptic ulcer*" has started to heal. Debra asked, "Ulcer? I don't have an ulcer. But, Mom, do you remember when Jeremy was three years old and got so sick, and we never knew he had pneumonia? Maybe that's the same thing. Maybe I had this virus and never knew it." Debra was given a special diet to follow. When she read it, she laughed. It was nothing different than what she been eating anyway, so no big changes in her diet. She ate healthy food items and always saw to it that Jeremy did, too. She is so hungry for something solid to chew on, but "Jerrrry, I can't have KFC fried chicken or spicy pizza!" Jerr told her, "But I love you, anyway."

She can't lie here anymore. A CT scan was performed. The doctor gave her meds to fight the infection. She has lacerated rings, needs an all liquid diet. She WANTS MEAT, or to go to a Chinese restaurant or even McDonald's. "I'm so hungry, Mom. The doctor reported there's a virus in my stomach, in the duodenum*." She was given Pepcid AC. It's hard to swallow, and about 6:45-6:50 p.m., the doctor came in to see her and stated she could be discharged. She was ready!

"Debra, let's talk about how we're going to pay for this hospitalization. Could you find out who I contact?"

5/3/09, Sun. —

Debra is feeling better. She is on the prescribed pills and will keep to her diet.

5/5/09, Tues. —

We think the weather has finally straightened out, and it is beautiful. Debra sits outside and then works on her little garden.

5/12/09, Tues. — En route to New York from Florida

There were phone calls with Debra, and when we arrived, we ran to each other with smiles, hugs and kisses. Later, we made arrangements to go out to dinner — an enjoyable time.

5/31/09, Sun.

I attended my church at St. Gregory the Great, a dynamic, spiritual church with a great priest, Father Joe, numerous ministries, a café, a Catholic store and a top notch school.

That evening, to celebrate our anniversary on June 1st, we went to the Grapevine Restaurant with our favorite neighbors, Lew and Sandra.

6/1/09, Mon. —

"Happy Anniversary, Mom & Jerr. I love you." The card she sent us: "Happy Anniversary, Mom and Dad.... patience...guidance... understanding....love...support. A day doesn't go by without the thought of how much it's meant to have parents like you. You're the best and I love you with all of my heart. Love & hugs, Debra, Donna, Jeremy.

(All of Debra's envelopes to us had mini-red hearts raining down from her name in the return address to our names. Even before opening the envelope, it brought smiles to our faces. She never forgot any holiday or occasion to send a card.)

(Jerr's friend, Dr.Pedro, and his wife, Nancy, had come in from Ohio, and we invited them to a gourmet luncheon served in the country under white tents. After a stroll through the hillside gardens and the gift shops, we returned home. A very relaxing afternoon.)

Debra received a call from a Medicaid person referred by the hospital. This person told her "Don't go to apply for food stamps today; if you wait until June 15, you will get two month's worth." *Food stamps?* "Why would I be getting food stamps, Mom?"

She had quite a delay getting her birth certificate from Colorado last October and other documents that had been requested. Then in January, she heard from Medicaid that although she had been informed to send them $17, they wanted 75 cents MORE. She had to go out and send a money order for 75 cents!

Two weeks later, Medicaid stated that Debra had to wait another 45 days because it was too early. She was being asked for more and more documentation. Finally Medicaid stated that her bank statement stated that she had a $25,000 annuity in her name! "WHAT? From where? Never have I had more than what was necessary

to cover my bills and never have I been aware of this money!"
When she asked her employer about that item, they told her that
"Corporate" had just put that amount in there to show a "distribu-
tion" on the records, but she doesn't have access to the funds nor
will she ever have access to those funds. So now she was informed
it would be 3-4 weeks before they can take it off! Something is very
funny there.

6/15/09, Mon. —

Plans for Debra's birthday lunch at the Cheesecake Factory were
changed because Donna wanted to attend and she found out she
was working on the 28th. She asked if maybe we could wait until
she's off on a Friday or the weekend that she doesn't work. Debra's
fiancée, Chris, had to work.

Debra said: "Mom, it's OK if it's even after the 4th of July! 🕯️🕯️
Are we still going to the river on the 4th of July for the fireworks?
(*Yes, as usual.*) "We can pretend the fireworks are for my birthday if
we haven't celebrated it yet!"

Personal: Chris' son borrowed Debra's phone charger and her
phone was dead. She had the rugs cleaned because of the boys and
dog; planted the vegetable garden; painted the front door and the
metal wrought iron gate Chris had made. By the time she feeds the
boys; does the laundry; picks up Jeremy (25 miles away) and back,
she runs out of time to celebrate, anyway.

6/20/09, Sat. —

Debra came to stay with us and wanted to go to Bed Bath &
Beyond to get Jerr a Father's day gift she had seen — a trunk
organizer. She always gave cards to Jerr for Father's Day, always
cutesy ones or with little jokes that he loved. She said Jeremy was
asking when they could go to Florida again — and we were laughing. 🕯️🕯️

6/26/09, Fri. —

Shopped at the local pharmacy for Debra's personal items, lipstick, lotion, and birthday cards.

7/3/09, Fri. —

Finally, we were able to celebrate Debra's birthday! She's a Cancer and a moon child. Donna had the day off work and the five of us had dinner at The Cheesecake Factory at the Walden Galleria Mall. Jeremy ordered his usual mini-sliders, and he and I shared the appetizer since you get six of them. Not only did we have dinner, most of which everyone took home, but then ordered their yummy desserts, so huge, we shared them among all of us!

Our card to Debra: *For my beautiful Daughter, Debra. I looked at you today and saw the same beautiful eyes that looked at me with love..... when you were a baby. I looked at you today and saw the same beautiful mouth that made me cry when you first smiled at me..... when you were a baby. It was not long ago that I held you in my arms long after you fell asleep, and I just kept rocking you all night long,*

I looked at yesterday and saw my beautiful daughter....no longer a baby but a beautiful person with a full range of emotions and feelings and ideals and goals. Every day is exciting as I continue to watch you grow and I want you to always know that in good and in bad times, I will love you and that no matter what you do or how you think or what you say you can depend on my support, guidance friendship and love every minute of every day. I love being your mother. By Susan Polis Schultz

Personal: Donna is a creative, talented person. She's worked as a secretary (taking after me?), but has had other interesting, high-activity jobs as well like Activities Director for a resort in Arizona, then at a nursing home in Niagara Falls; office manager for a blue ribbon cleaning service; as desk clerk for hotels, and at an outlet mall. With the exception of her job in Arizona, none of these jobs, however, provided her with medical insurance coverage.

7/4/09, Sat. —

Jerr and I left early for the Niagara River for the fireworks and found a super location. Debra and Chris met us. After the spectacular display, we had dinner at 11:00 p.m. at The Olympic. Jerr and I looked at each other and said, "Golly, we haven't been out this late for months!" Everybody was laughing. ⏏ ⏏

7/14/09, Tues. —

"Mom, are we going to Canalfest?" (*Of course, sweetheart, just like we do every year!*)

Personal: Debra's receiving a form from the State Insurance fund hopefully means that she is going to get her mileage check delayed from the time of the accident four years before. She is due thousands of dollars! Jeremy's father, Phil, picked Jeremy up on Saturday to take him fishing. The next day, Debra took Jeremy and a friend to Snowfest for ice skating (in the summer!). They go to the Reservoir there for sledding in the winter, too. The Reservoir was one of their favorite places. There's a beautiful cemetery at the base of the hills. But in July at Snowfest, they said it was kind of hard to skate on the "plastic". Jeremy received As and Bs on his report card; she was thrilled.

7/15/09, Wed., 11:00 a.m. — @ E/R, NFMMH

Debra has been in the hospital all night with excessive uterine bleeding. She was given a shot which was injected slowly. It was progesterone⋆ to stop bleeding; has had no answers yet. She has also received a referral to a gynecologist, Dr. Bee, as soon as her insurance company approves it.

She laughed and said: "Jerrrrry, it's your tax dollars at work." (*She loved to roll the rs in his name.*) Jerr told her, "The heck with that, let's get you well." She was given Motrin 500 mg. a pain shot and blood work. A doctor asked if she had had a miscarriage. "NO! Never."

7/25/09, Sat. —

She's been given prescriptions; antibiotic 3x a day, Prilosec, and more progesterone. With the referral to the gynecologist, hopefully, she'll get answers about what is wrong with her. She was laughing and told Jerr: "I can move to Florida now and line up all my little pills. Never in my life have I had to take any medication. I'm like my Mom!"

7/29/09, Wed. —

Debra and Jeremy stayed with us this weekend; we had dinner at the Buffalo Brew Pub. Jeremy was amazed at the crunch-crunch on the floor from peanut shells. The Pub has self-serve baskets of popcorn and peanuts the shells which are swept off on the floor! He was reluctant to do it, then he looked around, he saw everybody doing the same thing. "This is neat, Mom," he told Debra.
🏆🏆

7/30/09, Thurs. —

We took Debra to our local pharmacy to pick up some of her medicines.

8/2/09, Sun —

At church, I revert to the time-old traditions of our Catholic Church, saying The Lord's Prayer, *Our Father, who art in heaven*..... and the Hail, Mary, *full of grace*..... and asked for petitions for Debra that we learn about her medical condition, and that it being a treatable minor setback.

8/3/09, Mon., 9:15 a.m. —

Debra's appointment with the gynecologist. The doctor couldn't even perform the Pap smear*, Debra was screaming in pain, and he could not even insert the instrument to take the smear. Later, he told Debra she had to have a hysterectomy* immediately.

8/19/09, Wed. —

We attended Erie County Fair with Debra and Jeremy; had a great but long day. Jeremy loved the police dog exhibition with the police and firemen and how the men could rappel the rock wall. He's always said he's going to the Police Academy when he graduates and then see if he can enter the Green Berets. (*His desire since he was 10 and he and Debra lived on Grand Island. He would play among the bushes and trees, and he and his friend would pretend to be the good guys hiding or searching for the bad guys. With the woods and the stream, it was a perfect place for boys to play.*) At the Fair, we lunched on our favorite foods and then much later had dinner at the famous Chiavetta's Chicken.

8/22/09, Sat. —

Debra was very quiet at dinner at the Super Fuji buffet, until she opened her fortune cookie and it brought a smile to her face, "Happiness measures a person's real worth!" ⚓ ⚓

(*In February 2012, I found this little paper strip in her wallet.*)

8/28/09, Fri. —

We bought lots of school supplies for Jeremy; then to an office supply store to get his favorite pens with the cushioned tip which he prefers.

9/3/09, Thurs. @ NFMMH —

Debra's surgery is scheduled today. She has had a "flu" all week; she's been in bed, thought it was the rain, has been drinking Gatorade. She didn't want us to take her but wanted Chris to be with her; he took the day off work and because she has to be at the hospital by 6:00 a.m. and didn't want us getting up at the "crack of dawn". They live five minutes away from the hospital, and we are an hour away, she said. The surgery is scheduled for 10:00 a.m. Jeremy has the day off school, he may be there, too; he knows she is having surgery, but Debra was concerned that she didn't know how she was going to feel, and she didn't want him to see her in pain.

She doesn't understand why with the small amount of food she's eaten that she has been constipated. She didn't want to go for surgery like that. When she finally had a bowel movement, a big blood clot came out; she was afraid that the surgery would be postponed if she was bleeding or if she told the doctor about the "flu". She has been taking acetaminophen (aspirin). I asked her if she didn't think the doctor should be informed as to what's been going on with her? "No, Mom, I just want to get it over with. Anyway, the doctors will make me as comfortable, and I will get pain meds and everything will be OK. And I'll let you know what's happening, but I don't want you guys to see me like this. I'd rather be miserable in private!" "And, Debra, I feel we should be there with you, but like it or not, we respect your reasoning."

I sat on pins and needles the rest of the day, sitting by the phone, not wanting to use it in case she called. I imagined all sorts of things like the surgery being postponed after all, like they couldn't do it, like there was a problem, and all the images a mother has for a daughter going through this.

Finally, Chris called us in the afternoon and said that the surgery was completed. He had been with her in recovery and until she was transferred to a private room. He was leaving to get his boys dinner.

(We asked if we could come to the hospital and he told us that Debra doesn't really want any company during this time; she will call as soon as she can.)

9/4/09, Fri. @ NFMMH —

Debra called late afternoon; she has been screaming in pain. The nurses said she has been given all the pain meds that were ordered but would contact the doctor again. **By that evening**, she was given pain meds, that helped immediately. But I'm wondering why the horrendous delay? During the night, her IV was taken out, and the next day she was again screaming in pain with no meds. Finally when the doctor came in, he noticed that she hadn't had a bowel movement and immediately ordered a suppository* for her and half hour later, she had relief. So they had been giving her pain meds but it was the b/m that was pushing on her stitches from the inside! I told her I wanted to be with her, and she said, "No, Mom, I have to go through this myself and I really don't want any company. If I'm miserable, I really don't want anybody here." I said, "Debra, I should be with you." She said, "I know, Mom, but I'm going to be OK." *(We love you, sweetheart.)* "I love you two, too." *(That was her special saying to us and always made us laugh.)* More phone calls back and forth and she seemed to be settling down and sounded more comfortable. I called late evening and there was no answer.

9/6/09, Sun. —

Debra is discharged at 9:00 a.m. We were there to pick her up. Her Discharge Medication Reconciliation Report stated, "Continue Ferrous Sulfate*, 325 mg, once daily, and ibuprofen, new: hydroquinone* 7.5 mg/APAP 500 mg, one every six hours as needed for pain, Lortab, 7.5/500 mg, 1-2 pills every six hours as needed for pain, and to discontinue: ketorolac*, metoclopramide*, Hydromorphone* 2 mg (Dilaudid*), hydrocodone 7.5 mg/APAP 500 mg and continue ibuprofen." *(What were these medications?)*

We wanted to bring Debra back to our home, but she said she would prefer to recover at Chris' house. She was barely walking and didn't even want to go for breakfast. She was very quiet and said she was tired. We stopped at Walgreen's across the street from the hospital to pick up the pain meds which the doctor prescribed. The pharmacist stated they didn't have them but they would call her when it was ready. *(What?!)* They never called; the line was always busy. She was in so much pain and waiting for pain meds; it seemed like an eternity and no call or no answer. We offered to take her to another location or another pharmacy, but she told us if they would have been able to locate this medication, the pharmacy would have done that. She was very uncomfortable. She called the doctor's office and the answering service called him late on Sunday. He had phoned the prescriptions into the pharmacy, but he called them again. She's in so much pain. Debra called the pharmacy again and was told, "No, we don't have them!" She was left on the phone for over five minutes. I called Walgreen's and could not get through. We were ready to drive to Niagara Falls and sit at the pharmacy until she had them. Wouldn't a pharmacy who probably services most of the patients from the hospital have an inventory of needed meds? The doctor said the reason for the pain meds is that gas makes the pains worse; she also has pain from the anesthetic, which causes additional gas in stomach which pushes against the stitches! All she can eat is yoghurt. Still no relief. Hard to believe.

10:00 p.m. Sun. —

Debra finally got her pain meds and Chris picked them up! She had been all day without relief.

9/7/09, Mon., Labor Day, about 3:30 p.m. —

Debra received a call from her gynecologist's nurse that the doctor wanted to see her immediately the next morning at 8:00 a.m. at the hospital. Debra called to tell us of the message. I went ice cold when I heard about the doctor's call. "Mummy, do you think something's wrong?" She started crying and I was crying, too. I said, "I think so, sweetheart, but whatever it is, we'll face it and go step-by-step. We'll be there." *(Jerr just hugged me. I told him that Debra never cries, is very staunch about everything, just doesn't cry. Never did I think that it was serious. Jerr and I tried to think of why he wanted to see her; never had I heard of, read about or talked to anyone in a similar situation. We were so naive. I couldn't even imagine why he wanted to see her, did the surgery have to be performed again, did something go wrong, what? We just didn't know.)*

9/8/09, Tues. —

Jerry and I left Williamsville at 7:00 a.m., picked Debra up in Niagara Falls at 8:00 a.m. for her 8:15 a.m. appointment with the doctor at the hospital. (*We thought this was a strange time because his office doesn't open until 9:00 a.m.*)

Debra was called into the exam room, and she turned and asked me to accompany her. There was a nurse present with the doctor. There he said, "Well, Debra, I have bad news; I guess you guessed from the call yesterday. In all my years of practice, I have never had to tell a patient this before. If I had known what I would find, I would have never scheduled the hysterectomy."

He proceeded to tell her she had **ascending cell cervical cancer*!** When he was sewing the cervix, it was falling apart and wouldn't hold the stitches; he put a rush on the pathology report and that is what it revealed. The rest of the discussion I heard as if I had cotton wrapped around my head. I stopped thinking, I stopped feeling, I was just numb. I looked at Debra sitting on the examination table and she just had a little smile on her face. She was staring at the doctor. Did she comprehend?

He told us she is being referred to Dr. LaiLai at Roswell Park Cancer Institute (RPCI) in Buffalo, NY, where she'll probably have to have radiation. Debra asked, "How long is that going to take?" The doctor stated, "You are not going to have a good year." We asked if it was treatable and he responded yes. Debra continued to smile and asked, "Am I going to lose my Farrah Fawcett hair do?" Dr. Bee didn't answer but stated that he would contact Dr. LaiLai's office and get Debra an appointment. I asked for a copy of the report to give to our oncologist friend. The doctor asked us to wait in the waiting room until he was able to print the report. The doctor asked us to wait in the waiting room until he was able to print the report.

Back in the waiting room, we told Jerr the news. Jerr held my hand. I was holding Debra's hand, she gave a couple of little gasps, cried a little, looked around at the other patients in the room and told me, "Boy, am I glad I had Jeremy. At least I have him. I would be devastated if I didn't have any children and was told this news. I can just imagine how a woman must feel with this news, Mom." When we received the copy of the Pathology Final Report collected on 9/4/09 it stated Uterus, supracervical hysterectomy: INFILTRATING MODERATED DIFFERENTIATE SQUAMOUS CELL CARCINOMA OF CERVIX. *(We knew not of what that meant — all I saw was the word "carcinoma".)*

We wanted to go for breakfast, but she stated that she would prefer to go home. I said, *"Debra, I don't want you to be alone, I would like to stay with you. Let's talk about this and make some plans."*

"Thanks, Mom, but we'll know more when I get that appointment. Right now, I'm in pain and I just want to go back to bed." After dropping her off with big hugs and I love you, I cried all the way home.

(Dear Lord, what must she have felt about this news, what must she have thought about Jeremy, and Chris and her plans for their life? Did she accept the news? Did she fully understand the news? I don't fully understand it so how could she? Did she think that it couldn't be true? Could we really believe that what the doctor stated that she could be cured? Rarely had I seen Debra in tears or sobbing. She was so staunch about things throughout her life, but did she go home now and cry? Cancer? That dreaded word — cancer. Please, God, wrap Your arms around my daughter and give her comfort for us.)

Later, the doctor's office called Debra and said they had not heard from Dr. LaiLai's office yet but that the appointment would probably be next Tues. 9/15/09.

Personal: Debra called Chris at work and told him the news but said she didn't want him to leave work to come home; they would talk when he gets home. She's not going to tell Jeremy anything yet. "He's 13. He will be 14 on 9/26/09 and just started high school and I don't think he needs this on his mind. The last thing I want is to have his school work affected. Mom, I've been sick since he entered his teens — what a bummer for him."

"Debra, how are you feeling, sweetheart? What are you thinking?"
"Mom, I just want to see what this is all about, do what they need me to do and get well. I don't want Jeremy to know anything yet. I really don't want to upset his life for nothing. He deserves to have his life." Once again and as always, her first thoughts were for Jeremy.

9/12/09, Sat. —

Back at the hospital for a CT scan.

Personal: Debra and Donna joined us for dinner at the Super Fuji buffet. We weren't in a very good mood, but we all put ribs (*which I don't eat meat*) on our plates so that Donna could have the bones for her little doggies (the Benzengy breed). She said it would be a TREAT for them since they don't get them often. She had brought a plastic baggie in her purse — only for the bones! She looked around and asked, "Do I look like little old ladies putting food in a purse to take home?" 🔨 🔨

9/13/09, Sun. — @ E/R NFMMH

Debra is in severe pain; feels like the stitches are pulling; doctors ordered blood work. The IV blew her arm up; the rubber strap was left on after the nurse left the room! A CT scan was performed and at 4:00, she was sent home; they stated they did not find anything.

9/14/09, Mon. —

The day before Debra's first appointment at RPCI, we arranged with Chris to meet at a hotel parking lot right off the Youngmann Expressway — the half way point between our houses — and he dropped Debra off. She stayed with us overnight. We had dinner at home and just talked and talked. When Debra went to bed, I put a sign of the cross on her forehead. She started laughing, "OMG, Mom, that reminds me of when we were young teenagers and you used to put crosses on our foreheads before we went out. That cross used to burn on our foreheads and we always felt your presence — not good when we were up to hanky panky!" *"Debra, you girls were never bad kids, just got into silly mischief with your friends."*

9/15/09, Tues. @ RPCI —

Debra's first appointment. After finding our way to this huge, intimidating complex covering several blocks, we parked and walked across the street. Her "appointment" spanned five hours while she was registered and transferred through four different departments and floors. All patients are given a green plastic ID card (like a credit card). After Dr. LaiLai's internal examination of Debra, we were called into a conference room with him and another woman, his secretary? He said he had to do the surgery again and then would begin her "treatment." *(I went cold. "Surgery again? It's not even been two weeks since her hysterectomy!" No answer, just a stare. "Why? What kind of surgery?" I had looked over at Jerr, and he was pale, just staring at the doctor. Later, he told me it reminded him of when his wife was diagnosed with breast cancer twenty years ago, suffering with chemo treatments for ten years until she lost her battle. I don't remember Debra asking any questions, she just looked at the doctor and then at us.*

Debra was given a Consent for Treatment and Release of Records and Payment Guarantee to sign. *(We had always offered to pay for the girls' food and their medical and were prepared to do just that now.)*

When the doctor left the room, that woman asked Debra if she had any questions, and she said, "Not really. I don't know what to ask or what I should ask. I don't know what's happening." The woman said Debra would hear from them.

(*I'm really bothered. She's having another major surgery so soon after her last one less than two weeks ago? What does he expect to find that the gynecologist didn't find? What "treatments." We were such novices in this whole experience. We were left with more questions than answers. I asked if we could call later when we had time to think and ask those questions. This was not offered as an option.*)

We stopped at Perkins, one of Debra's favorite places, where she ordered a BLT (always that or a turkey club). We talked about the surgery, and I asked her how she felt. "*Debra, are you sure you want to do this? Can't we explore other options? I don't know what to do. I don't know who to call.*" "Mom, I'm going to have to do what I have to do. What choice do I have?"

At home, we envelop Debra in our arms and just held on to her. I didn't want to let her go. All of a sudden, she took a big breath and gasped, "I have to breathe you guys!" We started laughing. She went into the den and took a nap watching TV. We met Chris at the hotel when he picked Debra up, spent a few minutes talking about she had been told, but Debra was anxious to get home.

(*Debra was given an At Home Medication Information List. It included: acetaminophen-propoxyphene* tablet, 625 mg-50 mg, one every four hours; ibuprofen tablet, 800 mg, one three times a day as needed. Then a Medication Reconciliation Medication History and Order Form which listed — acetaminophen-propoxyphene tablet, one every four hours; ibuprofen tablet, 800 mg, one three times a day as needed; Tylenol with codeine, #3 tablet 300 mg-30 mg, one every six hours as needed for pain.*)

(*When we returned home, I just sat and cried and cried and asked God, why, why, why? Jerr just held me, and I knew he felt the same about this girl he loved as much as I did.*)

9/16/09, Wed. — @ NFMMH

Debra is enduring the same routine tests, the same story, and being told they couldn't find anything. Upstate Pharmacy delivers Hydromorphone 2 mg.

9/24/09, Thurs. —

Debra and Jeremy spend the day with us and at the pool. We had sandwiches and fruit for lunch; they swim some more, shower and we go out for dinner.

9/26/09, Sat. — Jeremy's birthday.

Debra and Jeremy went to their favorite park. They love nature and they walk and walk in the woods, sit under a tree and talk for over three hours. When Debra told him she had to go to the hospital again, Jeremy asked all kinds of questions, and Debra gave him information that she knew he could understand and handle. She has such intuition when it comes to Jeremy and his feelings. We celebrate his birthday out for dinner. He doesn't want a birthday cake, just a quiet, comfortable time with his Mom and us. He loves his birthday presents and gift cards. However, later, we did have Jerr's special cupcakes — Jerr taught them to pull the top half of the cupcake with the frosting, turn it over and make a cupcake "sandwich" with the frosting in the middle. Jeremy laughed and couldn't believe Jerr. He raised that eyebrow of his because he thought Jerr was joking with him again, but he loved it when he tried it. Forever after, that's how we ate our cupcakes — Jerr's way! Before Jeremy would pull his cupcake apart, he would look over at Jerr with that eyebrow lift and a smile, and we would all laugh.

9/30/09, Wed. —

Debra has been informed that she was being admitted to RPCI on 10/7/09. She told me, "Oh, — what would you say, Mom, 'Thanks be to God. It wasn't scheduled before Jeremy's birthday!' "

10/6/09, Tues. —

Chris dropped Debra off at the hotel parking lot and she stayed with us overnight. We talked this whole situation over. I was very nervous. Another surgery?

10/7/09, Wed. — Surgery @ RPCI.

We left Williamsville at 8:00 a.m. arriving at the hospital at 9:00 a.m. Debra went through the check-in process. There was a truly lovely person who took care of her at the Registration desk. We then were directed up to the surgical floor. Debra was taken to a pre-surgery room at 11:00 a.m. We saw Dr. LaiLai, then several nurses; then finally she was ready at 11:30. We were informed the surgery would be approximately two hours.

Jerr and I spent the time at the cafeteria for lunch, sitting at the mezzanine, listened to the lovely piano music by a performer in the lobby. We walk around the complex, we read notices, went for coffee, read magazines. Two hours came and went, then three hours, and I was just so nervous. We didn't know where to go, we didn't know who to call to ask what was happening. I was terrified.

At 3:00 p.m., FOUR HOURS LATER, Dr. LaiLai came out and standing in the waiting room in front of everyone, he told us the operation was done. He said the surgery was a success with the cervix and lymph nodes in her groin, however, he found cancer in her stomach and a little further up (*I asked where — her lungs? Where?*) No answer, but he continued that she is going to have to have chemotherapy* but that they'd let her recover from the surgery first. He said she would be taken to the 6th floor at 3:30 p.m., and we should go up there at 4:00 p.m. and we could see her.

I called Donna and left a short message on her phone. Chris arrived at the hospital after work as arranged and we told him the news. We were all hugging and crying.

At 4:00 p.m. —

We all went up to the 6th floor and were informed that she wasn't there yet to wait in the Waiting Room. The girl at the desk was not very friendly or helpful! TWO AND A HALF HOURS LATER — at 6:30 p.m., Debra was finally brought up, and we saw her briefly. She was hooked up to IVs, oxygen, a drainage tube, staples and bandages on her belly, and two lines of pain medication which she was told she could control herself — pain meds and morphine. She could "administer it every six minutes". (*Not so we learned later.*) Her nurse, Merry, was a lovely, superior nurse. She told us Debra would be sleeping most of the evening and next day, that as it's been a long day, we should go home and rest. I didn't want to leave Debra. But Merry told us we could call later than evening and she would inform us of Debra's condition. We were comfortable with that, and we all left about 8:00 p.m. We talked to Chris and we were crying again. Later when I did call, Merry said Debra was still asleep and I asked her to tell Debra that we had called.

10/8/09, Thurs. @ RPCI.

Late morning, I called the nurses' station and Debra's nurse, Lee, (we didn't like her as much) informed me Debra's been sleeping most of day, drinking a little; has severe pain. If she could, I asked her to tell Debra that we would be there shortly and asked what she was being given or her pain, Lee stated that Debra was "comfortable". (*How could she be comfortable if she had severe pain? I wondered.*)

1:00 p.m. —

When Jerr and I arrived at the hospital, we passed three nurses talking at the desk. They saw us pass but didn't say anything to us. When we were approaching Debra's room, we could hear her screaming before we reached her door and found that the door was closed shut. When we entered the room, Debra was writhing in pain and crying. When she saw us, she put her arms up and said "Mommy, Mommy, help me, it hurts so much, what's wrong?" I ran out to the nurses' station and said "My daughter is screaming in pain — who's her nurse?" The nurses all looked at what I assumed to have been the call board. One of them came around the desk and said, "There's been no call from her." She followed me back to Debra's room. In the meantime, Jerr was with Debra and holding her hand.

When I went back in to Debra's room, I was looking all over her bed for the call button. It was nowhere to be found. I asked "Where is her call button?" We were looking all around for it. I finally found it on the floor in the corner behind and underneath the cabinet! Debra couldn't even reach the phone, or the cabinet which was pushed back into a corner, least of all the call button!

I again asked the nurse, "Who did this and who was the last person in here and who closed her door tight so she couldn't be heard asking for help?" No answer. The nurse told me Debra had been given a pain pill at 9:00 a.m. (*Excuse me — A pain pill, A pill — after her second major surgery in a few weeks- A pain pill and now it was 1:00 p.m.! I was furious, but I know Debra doesn't like a fuss being made, so I kept quiet. She says the staff find a way of retaliating when complaints are received or patients create a problem. I did question the nurse about the pain meds.*) The nurse stated that the doctor had ordered that Debra was supposed to be given the pill every six hours. (*Obviously, it wasn't sufficient! We were furious. Jerr and I just looked at each other.*) I bent over and hugged what I could touch of Debra — my beautiful daughter, and I was sick to my stomach — what did we just agree to? I was crying; I couldn't believe what had just happened to my daughter.

At 1:45 p.m., the nurse came in, said she had called the doctor who ordered Percocet* which she had ready in her hand and injected it into Debra's IV line. Right after that, within about 20 minutes, Debra became comfortable, and we could just see the pain ebbing away from her. She smiled at us, she reached out and held our hands, but said the top of her thighs were so painful, she couldn't find a comfortable position. Can I massage them? Can I ask the nurse? I called the nurse again and asked that question. She responded it was from the surgery. (.......AND?) *But Debra gave us a weak smile and said, "Mom, it reminds me of when you made us take dance lessons and every Saturday, we were complaining that our legs hurt, that our thighs were sore, and that.... boo hoo, boo hoo, we didn't want to go to dance lessons, so we quit. Years later, I found out that Donna wanted to continue the lessons! Oh, just great!)*

At 5:45 Debra was given two 7.5 mg Gas-X* for gas.

It was about this time that Dr. LaiLai stopped across the room standing between the door and her bed asking her how she was and when she began to respond, he turned around and left. He was accompanied by a dozen other people (interns?) standing out in the hallway. When they all left, Debra said they all just stared at her — she felt like a specimen. *(Hello, there's a human being lying on this bed.)*

(On our way home that evening, we stopped at Wegmans for a floral arrangement. Debra loved it when we put it on her cabinet the next morning. She gave us a huge smile and later told me the aroma was so comforting because it reminded her of her gardens. Debra had designed a beautiful garden in Chris' tiny front yard and she said people coming from a nearby bed and breakfast inn to the Falls would stop and take pictures and talk to her if she was on the porch. She also designed other gardens for people.)

10/09/09, Fri. — @ RPCI.

Today the catheter was removed; she's still in severe pain and complains about her upper left chest, why, she asked when she thought the surgery was lower. *(I asked. The nurse said she'd check but we did not receive an answer.)* We tried to make Debra feel better; asked the nurse about the pain and pain meds. She said she would call the doctor.

(He never got back to us while we were there. We left about 6:30 p.m. I called the nurses station that evening and was informed that "Debra was sleeping and comfortable." In retrospect, I feel that I should have stayed with Debra — not to interfere but to let her know that if she needed help, there's someone to assist in getting it. Yes, those were my feelings, but I was reminded of Debra's need for privacy.)

10/10/09, Sat. — @ RPCI.

The IV tubes were removed from her hand (wrist) and right arm, and she felt much better. We hugged her and she smiled at us. She told us not to come to the hospital the next day until she calls us as she thinks she's being discharged but doesn't know at what time. She will call us and by the time we get there, she will be ready for discharge. *"Sweetheart you don't need help in dressing and packing your things?"* "Mom, I can try to manage, even it takes me a long time."

10/11/09, Sun. —

Debra discharged from RPCI at 12:20 p.m. The drainage tube was removed, she still had pain in upper left chest; a different nurse said that was because of the clamps. *(So, OK, that's all we needed to know previously, but clamps?)*

Debra had called and said that depending on the time of her discharge, that Chris wanted to pick her up from hospital since he worked just around the area and it was on his way home. As it was, he picked her up at 3:30 p.m. She called us when she got home — tired, in pain, but so glad to be home.

(Debra was given a Medication Reconciliation Medication History and Order form. It included:

acetaminophen-propoxyphene tablet, 325 mg-50 mg, one every four hours; ibuprofen tablet, 800 mg, one three times a day as needed.)

10/12/09, Mon., Columbus Day —

Jeremy spent an hour with Debra in Niagara Falls. She showed him her stitches with the staples; told him the doctor had to take something else out and the reason he couldn't come to see her when he was in Niagara Falls was that she was in a Buffalo hospital. She has to go back to the doctor's office, be put on a machine of some kind to take care of a few more things so she gets well. He was OK with that explanation.

She told me: "Mom, of course, if I was told I had six months to live, of course, I'd tell Jeremy. But I haven't been told that. How do I know what to tell him?" (*We are aware that RPCI is known for telling a patient the truth. My sister's best friend had been referred to RPCI and was told she only had two weeks to live and it was only one week before she was gone.*) "Mom, I don't want him to go through what Phil went through when he lost his mom when he was 16. It affected his schoolwork. Later, when he was elected Most Valuable Football Player and received honors at graduation, they didn't mean a thing to him. I don't want that for Jeremy."

"Mummy, I can't clear my throat, probably because of the tube they put down my throat." She was crying all day, every half-hour, she said. ♀

(*Tube? What tube. All I could think to tell her was that it perfectly normal to have these emotions. Her body had received a shock — a second one in that many weeks. Chris didn't know what to do; I told her to tell him, just hold me, Chris. But where do we get information, who do we talk to, how can I help my daughter? I curled up in a ball on the bed. I could feel her pain and I didn't know what to do.*)

10/13/09 - Tues. — Niagara Falls

10/14/09 - Wed. — Niagara Falls —

Personal: Ginny and boys went to Chris' house with a cheesecake for Chris' birthday and stayed until 9:30 p.m. Debra was in severe pain, and Chris couldn't get her out of bed. He called us and said there was no way he could get her up and drive her to Williamsville to stay with us. We told him, No problem, Chris.

Also, my sister, Erma, who lives in Colorado sent me an email from the Rocky Mountain Cancer Centers.

©LOVE HEALS

> The Power of LOVE is Hard to Ignore

> Love. It makes hearts grow fonder, blood move faster, and creates that never-want-to-live-without-it feeling for everyone it encounters. Surprisingly, love also has an unmistakable therapeutic power. It has been scientifically proven to aid healing and help improve the lives of people, animals, and plants alike. And with the help of our experienced doctors and caring staff, it's now making its way into the hearts of every patient at Rocky Mountain Cancer Centers.

Personal: Erma and Lou's first son, Aaron, was diagnosed with leukemia at the age of 22 while he and his wife were expecting their first child. He passed away two weeks after his daughter was born; he was able to hold her and leave her with a picture together with her dad. During the days and long nights that Erma sat with her son through his pain, his tests, his improvements and his devastating illness, she would send daily emails about the events and her feelings. Since then Erma has been very involved in cancer-related activities and events. She once told me, "A mother should never have to bury their child." Little did I know what that would come to mean!

10/15/09 - Thurs. -12:55 p.m. appointment at RPCI, Amherst Clinic —

Chris got Debra up at 8:30 a.m., then drove in the opposite direction to Lewiston to pick up Ginny, his mother, returning to Niagara Falls to get Debra. They all drove to Williamsville to drop Debra off to us before taking his mother to the Sheridan Drive surgical center for minor knee surgery at 10:30 a.m. God bless, Chris, what a caring, giving person he is! Nothing is a problem to him.

At Amherst, Debra's staples were removed and bandaged up again; she was in severe pain; complained of pain in her upper left chest.

At 2:30 —

After a long wait, a chemo nurse came in and wanted to explain everything to Debra and us. It all sounded so complicated, dozens of pamphlets, instructions and meds; I could not even follow her, totally confusing, all the terms and phrases thrown at us. We were numb. Debra was very impatient to get out of there because of the pain and said "Just give me something I can read at home." She did not want to hear all the medical terms this nurse was rattling out to us.

Debra came home with us, ate a little soup and a turkey sandwich, took her meds, went to her bedroom and fell asleep.

While she slept, I picked up the literature and read and read and read. OMG, how was she going to do all this? How could we help her? Jerr and I discussed having her stay with us if we could convince her. I made a list of all the anti-bacterial wipes and other things she was going to need. We separated her towels and wash clothes and sponges. She was going to need as sterile an environment as possible.

Around 5:30 p.m. —

I heard Debra rush to the bathroom, then she called out for me and through the door, she said she was bleeding all over her underpants and her slacks. (*The underpants were new ones without an elastic waistband which did not hurt her around the incision.*) She said there was such a smell and that she needed wings. (*Wings? She needs wings?* "*Mom, Wings are sanitary pads for menstrual periods! Oh.*) Wandering around the grocery store, finally found them and got her two large packages. I offered to take her to the hospital next door to us or to call Dr. LaiLai. She said no, she'll handle it. Besides what will another hospital know about the treatment she has had or needs? She asked for cleanser and paper towels and disinfectant and spent a hour cleaning my bathroom. (*Wasn't necessary, sweetheart.*)

6:30 p.m. —

Meanwhile, Chris was on his way to pick her up at our place. Debra was very short with me, with Jerr and then Chris. I knew she was worrying about what had just happened and the pain she has. I told Chris you can tell she's nearing the time for her next pain med. He said, "I let it roll off my head. She doesn't bother me." What a special guy. They left about 9:30 p.m.; we gave them a roasted chicken to take home.

Debra: "I love you two." "We love you, too, Debra."

10/16/09, Fri. @ home in Niagara Falls.

Debra's in a lot of pain, she eats a little; drinks a little; then falls back to sleep. She'll call us when she can. In the meanwhile, Chris and I will continue to keep in contact with each other.

Upstate delivers Dexamethasone* 4 mg, Prochlorperazine* 1 mg, Emend* 125-80 mg.

10/17/09, Sat. —

Debra and Donna were supposed to get together to bake and decorate a cake for Chris' birthday. It didn't happen. She was so sick. One of Debra's talents was cake decorating and making specialty cakes.

10/18/09, Sun. —

Again, no cake baking — Chris said Deb was so sick. I asked if there was something we could do and he said not right now, but I'll let you know.

As family and friends learned of Debra's diagnosis, they began calling, sending greeting cards, or prayer cards. Everyone was absolutely wonderful and encouraging — all except for one callous person. Such a support system was so important to both Jerr, me and Debra and the rest of the family.

10/19/09 - Mon. —

A nurse practitioner from RPCI, Kris, called me looking for Debra. I called Deb's phone, then called on Chris's cell phone, and he said she was talking to someone from RPCI. Debra told Kris how sick she was, the trouble she was having and about the massive discharge which smelled like a "dead animal". Debra was keeping herself so clean; disinfecting herself as instructed; putting on clean clothes and when the wound started draining again; she could smell it. She also had what seems like be a hole at the bottom of the incision and that was draining, too. Kris said, "Debra, you need to go to the Emergency Room immediately!" There's no one in her office except Charron and her. Debra did not know who she was. Kris called me again to please let them know what the doctors in Niagara Falls find and how she's being treated.

Debra slowly got up and dressed, and Chris took her to NFMMH about 4:00 p.m. The NFMMH nurse called me at 5:30 p.m. and asked what kind of surgery had Debra had. At that time, we had not been told what kind of surgery only that it was abdominal. Debra remembered a term "vertical laparoscopy." I said I had never heard the term. (*A year later in 2010, we found out that her surgery in 2009 was for exploratory lap, radical trachelectomy*).

10:00 p.m. —

The nurse called and we were told Debra had bronchitis and a severe wound infection! She was given a large antibiotic pill and a prescription to be pharmacy-filled, and she was sent home.

She was crying and said, "Mommy, I can't take any more of this. In my whole life, I've never even had a cold."

In the meantime, I returned Kris' call from RPCI, spoke to her and reported Debra's symptoms, and what she had been told at the hospital. Kris said, "Yes, she needed to go to the E/R."

10/20/09 Tues., 7:00 p.m. —

Debra is feeling better already, sitting outside on their porch and enjoying the few Halloween lights they put up; it's real quiet. She said, "I think I'm going to have a talk with Phil and tell him what's going on and that he's got to step up to the plate and start bringing Jeremy to her in Niagara Falls. "I can't be driving from Niagara Falls to Buffalo like I have at all times of the year, even during blizzards to pick Jeremy up to spend time with me and then take him back. But I will, Mom, because it's never been a problem no matter how sick I've been or how horrible the weather is. Jeremy's my whole life." She doesn't want Jeremy to know anything yet.

Her stomach is getting a little softer; the right side is bigger than the left side, so all that stuff is coming out but yuk! She said Aunt Chickie called and left a message, but she couldn't call her back; she just didn't have the energy. (*Chickie is our nickname for my sister, Mary.*)

Debra wanted to take her car off the road and cancel the insurance for the months she won't be driving. Chris has paid the insurance and when he discussed it with the insurance company, the agent stated it would be more of a problem than leaving it on. It doesn't matter what she does with the car and insurance, just that Debra is paying for it and she's doing it in spite of having no income. (*We have been supporting her. Debra was always so proud that she was able to pay all her expenses on her income, care for Jeremy and still have fun times together.*)

(*Also, Chris had to go to Phil's house in Depew to move Debra's furniture; Phil wouldn't help because of a "bad back", just watched Chris do it. Chris said, "It doesn't matter, I'll do it. I'd do anything for her." Phil told Chris, "This is what she wants, so that's what it's going to be.........."*)

1:00 p.m. —

Tammy in Kris' office at RPCI called me; I informed her of Debra's symptoms, and she stated that the chemo treatment would be put on hold until she recovered. I asked her what kind of surgery Debra had undergone, and she said a **laparoscopy bilateral (upper covering of abdomen)**. (*When I found Debra's files in 2012, there was a surgical Patient Information Form which stated she was scheduled for: Exploratory lap, radical trachelectomy.*) (*Later, I looked it up and it is "laparotomy" — an incision in the stomach.*)

Debra was checked and the lymph nodes removed in her groin. The chemo is for cervical cancer precaution. Tammy asked what kind of meds Debra was given. I called Chris in Niagara Falls, he said she was given lung spray (Voltaren HFA), 90 mcg, 1-2 puffs as needed every 4 hours; the antibiotic is Sulfameth/Trimethoprim, 800 mg/160 tabs, count 20, twice a day until they are finished; and Tramadol*. Later, Tammy called back and said Dr. LaiLai wants to see Debra at RPCI in Buffalo on Thursday, 10/29/09; the schedule will be sent to me here in Williamsville.

(*On 10/21/09, Debra received prescriptions for: Oxycodone* 10 mg/*

APAP 5 mg [a narcotic used to relieve moderate to severe pain] (what was this about?); Polyeth glycol* 3350 NF Powder 255 gm (to control constipation); Sulfameth/ Trimethoprim 800/169 tabs (antibiotic combination used to treat or prevent infections; Tramadol 50 mg [an analgesic used to treat moderate to moderately severe pain]; and Ventolin HFA Inhaler 200 puffs [a bronchodilator used to treat or prevent the symptoms of asthma, emphysema, and other breathing conditions].)

10/28/09, Wed. evening —

Chris dropped Debra off and she stayed over with us. My friend, Sandra, and I went to pick her up. At 4:00 a.m., during the night she called me that she was very ill; she felt very warm. When I took her temperature, it was 103°! I gave her Bayer 400 mg aspirin, and one hour later, it broke her fever and she was perspiring and soaking wet. (*Good!*) I was still up so we got up, washed and changed clothing and bedding. At 10:00 a.m. the next morning, she came into the dining room, smiling and waving her hands at us saying the "Grateful Dead" is awake and living! Let's eat." ⚓ ⚓

1:30 p.m. We went to RPCI where she registered, had blood drawn (very poor technician!); then went to the 2nd floor GYN Clinic. The nurse said Debra had hives all over her body. Deb thought it was from using the antiseptic soap when she took a shower. The nurse said, "No, it's hives/allergy from the antibiotic." When she saw the name of the antibiotic, the nurse said it **contained sulfur** and in the future, Debra is to indicate that she is allergic to sulfur! The nurse will have the doctor order a different antibiotic and have it delivered to her home today.

A visiting nurse was ordered to go to her home every day to repack the incision as they did that day. The nurse said the incision was 1-½" deep and that it had to be cleaned out every day with saline and re-packed — with a long string with little cotton balls on them and inserted into the incision. She said there couldn't be any air pockets there because then the incision would have to be opened up again and "we don't want that, do we?" Then she put a large square padding on her stomach. They want to see her again next week; they will check the incision and take a chest x-ray.

Thursday evening — Debra couldn't stay over with us because her medicine was being delivered and the nurse coming to her home. Chris came over about 4:30 p.m. after work to pick her up.

We talked about the changing of the seasons, and all the beautiful leaves which had turned a brilliant gold, red, orange. Debra said she and Jeremy always loved walking in the woods during autumn when it was so quiet and there was only the sound of the rustling of the leaves under their feet. She laughed and said, "Remember when Jeremy was a little boy and you were picking him up at day care every day and he stayed with you until either I or Phil got out of work? He helped you rake your back lawn which was so huge it looked like a park. When you finished piling the leaves neatly by the tree, you said, 'Jeremy, let's jump in the piles.' You said he looked at you like you couldn't mean it. Then you jumped first and you guys spent the next half hour jumping and laying in the leaves and looking up at the sky and laughing. You finally came into the family room, and Jerr took one look at the two of you and asked, 'What in the world have you been doing?' You guys had leaves in your hair, on your clothes, on your shoes. But you were all laughing. And Jerr looked out the back door and the leaves were scattered almost where they were in the lawn, and he just shook his head." "I know, we had fun taking his bath that night before he was picked up and I soaked in my own bath later on."

"Mom, I also remember when you told Jeremy you were going to have a night picnic. Again, he looked at you like he didn't know what you were talking about — a night picnic? You went out in the back yard with a blanket, fruit and bottles of water and lay down on your backs looking at the night sky, the stars, the new moon just coming out, and he was asking you all kinds of questions. Later, he kept wanting to do it all the time and you explained that only when the stars and the moon were in place could you have a night picnic! But you had several night picnics." 🛶 🛶

"Debra, I also remember that you are a Moon Child, and we always promised to think of each other every full moon no matter where we were. I still do that." "I know, Mom, me, too."

Debra's Schedule

(This schedule would be repeated over her treatment period!)

DATE	DAY/ TIME	LOCATION	SCHEDULED PROCEDURE	NOTES	COMPLETED	NURSE
One week before chemo.			Call pharmacy for delivery of all meds.			
First day of chemo.			5-hours	One hour before: take Emend 125 mg		
2nd day of chemo.			Take at same time in morning.	Emend, 80 mg tablet AND Dexamethasone, 8 mg. (Decadron*) (2 tablets of 4 mg. each)		
3rd day of chemo				Emend, 80 mg tablet AND Dexamethasone, 8 mg. (Decadron) (2 tablets of 4 mg. each)		

4th day of chemo				Only Dexametha-sone, 8 mg (2 tablets of 4 mg each)	
IF NEEDED with or after EMEND is compl.				Compazine — one 10 mg. tablet every 6 hours IF NEEDED.	
10/29/09	Thurs., 1:30 p.m. 1:45 p.m. 2:00 p.m.	RPCI-Buffalo	Phlebotomy Unit Ground Floor GYN Clinic-Check-in (2nd Floor) GYN-Dr. LaiLai		YES

Additional Instructions:

Very important, drink eight (8) 8-oz (2 liters) glasses of water each day to prevent dehydration and keep your bowels moving and flush the veins. Increase juices, fruits, vegetables. She is to take her temperature. If 100.5°, it means you're anemic, if light-headed, dippy. If white blood cell count, highly susceptible to inflections.

OTC meds. —

Motrin, 400 mg every 6 hours AS NEEDED for leg cramping or joint pain.

Benadryl, 50 mg — may be used at bedtime to help you sleep.

Laxatives like: Smooth Move Tea, Pericolace, Milk of Magnesia — if you don't move your bowels in two days.

Blood tests need to be drawn **every** week on **non**-chemo weeks. Chemo causes a drop in blood counts.

White blood cells — fight infection

Hemoglobin — red blood cells carry oxygen in body

Platelets — help blood to clot and prevent bleeding.

10/30/09, Fri. 10:20 a.m. —

The antibiotic wasn't delivered yesterday; also that the Percocet has caused her finger tips to burn. She has taken ibuprofen 800 mg or Tylenol with codeine. I called RPCI, Kris, and left this message. Deb also said the visiting nurse had called and was coming at 10:30 p.m. for her daily visit. Deb was sitting shivering just thinking how gross it was going to be and didn't want to go through this "cleaning" again. She said when the nurse took out the cord, cleaned her belly and then reinserted it, it felt like a knitting needle being stuck in there (at the bottom of the incision). She was trying not to scream.

Upstate delivers Levaquin* 750 mg.

11/2/09, Mon. — To RCPI. Appt. with Dr. LaiLai.

Debra's infection has cleared; she was given a depraphrone* shot (progesterone) for hot flashes. Dr. LaiLai wants to start chemo treatments tomorrow. Finally left there at 3:30 p.m.

11/4, 5, 6/09 - Chemo Procedure: Cisplatin*

Debra's four hour treatment; chemo tends to sit in the kidneys
and that is not wanted, so she will be given Lasix (water pills).
She may develop neuropathy* which means numbness or pain
in feet or bottom of feet and her fingers and she is to let the
nurses know immediately. Cisplatin treats cancer of lung, ovaries,
bladder, testicles.

Decadron for nausea is a steroid; it tends to give a buzz, sleepless
nights; the cheeks may turn pink.

Constipation: Take Miralax, takes up to three days; do not leave
bowel movement more than two days, may be nausea in stomach.

Topotecan is a 30-minute infusion. It treats ovarian cancer
and small cell lung cancer; may cause constipation; call
them immediately.

Debra may develop mouth sores.

11/5/09, Thurs. —

We stopped at Panera's for lunch. Debra ordered her usual turkey
sandwich and Jerr his usual ham and cheese. We shared donuts,
and she and Jerr were fighting over the chocolate frosting left on
the slip of wax paper they use. 🍩🍩

11/5 to 15/09 —

Deb says she spent the time cleaning house, doing laundry, getting
paperwork organized and packing her case for the hospital.

11/16/09, Mon. —

Same routine, Chris drops Debra off, we pick her up and she
spends the night with us.

11/20/09

Upstate delivers Metoclopramide 10 mg.

11/17 - 18/09 - Chemo Procedure: Cisplatin

11/19 - 20/09 - Chemo Procedure Topotecan.

11/17/09, Tues. —

After Debra's five-hour chemo treatment, we take her to
Carrabba's Italian Grill. She loved it — the food, the service, the
fresh, crusty bread dipped in oil and herbs, the hot soup in a warm
bowl, the cold, crispy salad in a chilled plate, everything! And the
amount of food! We couldn't finish and had to take half home. Jerr
had ordered mussels and when he received his order, they were in
oil and garlic. He quietly mentioned he was a little disappointed
because he imagined the mussels in tomato sauce. The menu
didn't state that and on closer reading, it said oil and garlic. Oops.
However, the waiter must have heard his comment, and before we
knew it, a dessert had come to the table. When we had finished our
dinners and were awaiting the check, the Manager/owner came
over with a huge paper take-out bag for Jerr, and there it was — a
whole order of mussels in tomato sauce! He smiled, patted Jerr's
shoulder and said, "In the future if that's how you want it, just
order it that way — we make it any way you want!" The aroma
of the garlic, mussels and tomato sauce permeated the car! Debra
laughed, "See, all the gifts that are around us? Boy, I sure wish I
liked mussels." Jerr throws his arm up and told her "Well, you can
feel my muscles when we get home, girly." We laughed all the way
home -- with the aroma of garlic. We asked can you imagine if
we get into a car accident, what will we smell like! "Yup, we'll be
charged with SDI." "SDI?" "Smelling while driving!" Jerr grabbed
his bag: "As l long as I can bring my take-out bag to the hospital!"
More laughter at the image of the E/R with his take-out bag! 🛆🛆

11/19/09, Thurs. —

After Debra's chemo, we had breakfast/lunch at the Cracker Barrel. Debra was hungry for pancakes! During breakfast, Debra started laughing and nudged Jerr and said, "Jerrrrry, do you see how Mom cuts her pancakes? All in neat little rows and then little squares. You and I just dig in wherever. And when Mom eats corn — OMG, it's like the old manual typewriters, a row at a time to the end, ding, return, and start the next row-ding! You and I both eat the same, just dig and our cobs look a mushy mess and Mom's are real neat! *"Right, but doesn't mine look good from your angle, hmmmm?"* "Mom, you mean the eating angle — ours? 😄 😄 "Then have you seen how she eats waffles? All the little grids cut in squares and filled with syrup. *Well, guys, remember the time Debra shocked the waitress by asking for cold syrup when she brought warm syrup in the little bottles? The waitress just stood there, shocked, and said she has never had that request before from a customer. And Jerr always, always leaves two bites of food on his plate. Two bites. Why? OK, OK, so we all have our little quirks, let's eat!* "Mom. that's why me and Jeremy love Pop Tarts — *no fuss, no muss and ready in minutes!"* 😄 😄

Chris picked Debra up later and she went home.

11/20/09, Fri. —

Upstate Pharmacy delivers the doctor's prescription of Metoclopramide.

11/24/09, Tues. — My birthday.

Debra and I went shopping at Bon Ton as she needed a few new clothes due to the weight loss. We had so much fun, laughing at silly things. 😄 😄 Chris picked Debra up at 9:00 p.m.

11/24/09, Tues. — @ E/R NFMMH

Chris called us at midnight, Debra is on an IV; a CT scan showed a blood clot; it feels like the flu but she's not throwing up. She's hungry; can't get warm enough. Dr. Singh says her stomach is OK; her problem doesn't have to do with an infection. He may want to do more tests; she has diarrhea and that could be causing her pains. She has lung lesions and has been put on Prilosec. (*Lung lesions?*) He said did we know that Dr. LaiLai's wife is doctor, too?

12/1/09, Tues. —

I sit down to address the Christmas cards. We were so hopeful and also grateful that RPCI was accessible to us.

12/3/09, Thurs. —

I helped Debra write a letter to VESA as they want an update. This pertains to the 2005 car accident. She'll tell them about her status and that she is unable to go to school or work. In January, she's going to the attorney who helped Lisa with her Social Security case. She cried, she's angry, but it's time to move on.

Personal: Where's an Old Navy store? Maybe at the Eastern Hills Mall? She saw a hooded jacket with fur. She doesn't have a nice one. (*We found the store and bought it for her as a Christmas present.*)

Upstate delivers Emend 125-80 mg.

12/4/09, Fri. @ RPCI —

Debra signed a "Patient Consent For Use Of Tissue For Research" which stated: "Risks: The greatest risk to you is the release of information from your health records. We will do our best to make sure that your personal information will be kept private. The chance that this information will be given to someone else is very small. However, there is no guarantee that the privacy of your personal information can be absolutely protected.

"The results of research with these tissues may be presented at scientific meetings and published in medical literature; but in anything presented or published, it will not be possible to identify you as an individual. There are no additional costs to you or your insurance provider associated with your agreeing to allow your leftover specimen/tissue to be use for research."

This Consent gave RPCI permission to conduct research on her specimen(s)/tissue(s) for research to learn about, prevent or treat cancer or **cancer-related diseases**; to keep specimen(s) / tissue(s) for use in research to learn about, prevent or treat other diseases, **in addition to cancer**; and that RPCI staff may use her clinical data (not personal identifiers) associated with the specimen/tissue to do research.

I questioned Debra about this Consent, she stated, she didn't remember but that after her surgery someone had brought a form for her to sign. When we discussed it, she said, "What does it matter, Mom, maybe they can learn something to help someone else. What was going to be done with it (*the tissue*) — just throw it away? Maybe I can help somebody else — God knows, I feel people are not being helped to date (in having cancer.)"

12/7/09, Mon., 10:30 p.m. —

We met Chris at the hotel when he dropped Deb off for her overnight stay with us prior to her chemo treatment tomorrow.

She also requested her medical records from NFMMH. *(Never received them.)*

(Debra received her first 3-pill dosage of Emend, Compazine and Decadron. We noted the cost of over $500 for these three pills. This process was to be repeated every time she received a chemo treatment. We were so impressed by Upstate Pharmacy because no matter whether she was with us or at her father's or home in Niagara Falls, NY — this pharmacy never made a mistake in their delivery.

12/8 - 9/09 - Chemo Procedure: Cisplatin

12/10-11/09 - Chemo Procedure: Topotecan

12/8/09, Tues., 10:00 a.m. @ RPCI Amherst Center —

When we arrived, there was a small waiting room but in the treatment room, there was a circle of recliners with the nurses' station in the center. There was a small wall TV and a curtain if you wished privacy — otherwise, you saw and heard everything. We were offered juice, coffee, tea, hot chocolate and lots of pastries, cookies, cakes, or whatever treat was there that day. The patients and their family/friends could help themselves.

Debra had begun the regimen that she would follow throughout the entire treatment schedule — take the Emend pill before chemotherapy treatment, then take her anti-nausea pills (2) after her treatment; the nurse said it would give her energy — she might even want to clean the house (she waited for a groan from Debra, but Debra told her, "Oh, I love to clean the house; my house is really clean." (She talked non-stop for five hours until she went to bed. Whew! Jerr and I laughed but we loved it. 👍 👍

10:00-3:30 p.m. Debra's appointment.

She wanted to go the Anchor Bar (visible from the hospital) where the famous chicken wings were created. You walk in and the aroma of chicken wing sauce is enticing; we could hardly wait for our order. There are photos of famous celebrities, politicians, sports figures and others displayed on the walls. Jerr ordered an extra full order to bring home to put in the freezer — the aroma followed us all the way home!

Debra has reported to the doctor that she had severe pain on her fingertips on her left hand. He stated that was a side effect from the pain medication and that he could give her nerve pills, but the side effects would be worse than the pain itself; see if she can tolerate the pain. If not, call and he will give her something else. We soaked her hands in warm water to see if that would alleviate the pain.

12/9/09, Wed. @ at RPCI Amherst Clinic —

8:00 a.m. to 4:00 p.m. — Debra's chemo treatment. For lunch we ordered her an egg salad sandwich from the Grateful Deli in the building and then returned there to have our own lunch. When Debra was finished, we came home and she slept.

12/10/09, Thurs., 9:30 a.m. @ Amherst Center —

Debra was given her (2) anti-nausea pills. Debra has light brown hair which cascades down to her waist. Now it has started to thin and then fall out on gobs. We never mentioned it until one day she called and said her hair was all over her house, her bedroom, the bathroom, her car. Hair was flying out. She put a mesh cover over the drain in the shower. Her thinning hair clogged up the vacuum; it was wrapping around the vacuum cleaner coil. Chris had to use the shop vac, but he told her, "It doesn't matter, Deb." She became so upset about it, was sitting down and crying. Eventually, she only had a long strip of hair left at the nape of her neck. It had become matted because she could not reach it to comb it out. She tried tying it in a pony tail and wearing her knit skull cap. (*One year for Halloween, Chris had given them all the skull cap which glowed in the dark! It was a joke but eventually, Debra said it was the softest, most comfortable cap she had to wear. Nothing else we tried was as comfortable as this cap. So many times, I wanted to offer to comb the pony tail and untangle it, but her scalp hurt the one time I tried so we never mentioned it again. It broke my heart to see it, remembering her beautiful, soft, fragrant hair.*)

During one of her treatments at the clinic, the nurse saw the "pony tail" under her cap. The nurse flipped off, "Honestly, why don't you just cut it all off — just get rid of it!" Later, in the car, Debra was crying. "She doesn't understand; I've had my long hair for 48 years. I've never cut it. Jeremy used to hold on to it ever since he was born. His little hands would grab on and hold. He's never wanted me to cut it either. He loves my long hair." She continued to be very upset, crying, "Does anybody here (*at RPCI*) think about a person's feelings?" ♀ ♀

"Deb, you know what I was thinking? I'll cut my hair to match yours and we'll be like mother and daughter! I will do it. I really will."

"OMG, Mom, that's funny. I can just picture you without hair. I always loved it when I used to cut your hair. It felt so silky and smelled so good. And it all fell into place. When I was going to beauty school, I kept wanting you to come and be my model, but my instructors said, 'No, you have to learn and practice on hard-to-cut hair!' and I told them, "Well, that's not my Mom's!" ⚓ ⚓

"Debra, that's because with just a few snips, you made my hair to fall into place. It was amazing! People would ask me where I had my hair done and I would tell them, 'At home!' I was happy when you entered beauty school. I had wanted you girls to go to college, but the money wasn't there by then and I felt so guilty."

"Mom, we didn't want to go to college, at least I didn't, maybe Donna did. I wanted to work with my hands — like a hair dresser or landscaper — or pet groomer, something like that. I know if we had really wanted to go to college, you would have made it possible somehow. It was our decision. It was our choice. So there, big lady!"

After Debra's chemo, we had dinner at Perkins Restaurant. She and Jerr are now laughing because they both order the same thing every time! Debra has a turkey club sandwich and Jerr orders their grilled ham and cheese sandwich. ⚓ ⚓ Another topic they would always laugh about was birthmarks. I have a small, tan birth mark above my left knee; Jerr has one at mid-leg and so does Debra have a tan birthmark at mid-leg! She always said "Jerrrrry, are you sure you aren't my father?" He always tells her, "I would have been proud to be your father, sweetheart."

Later, she was feeling blue again. She called Chris to pick her up immediately but he had stopped after work with the guys for their annual lottery selection, but he told her, "Sure, OK, honey, I'll be there as soon as this is over." He picked her up at 9:00 p.m.

12/11/09, Fri. —

After her chemo treatment, Jerr and I had an appointment with our lawyer in Lancaster. Debra surprised us by saying that she wanted to meet with him, too. She wanted to prepare a will to have Jeremy and his trust fund administered by both of us. After we introduced her to David, she met privately with him. Later, we had "lundin" (what I call lunch and dinner) down the street at the Olive Tree. We talked about what she had decided, and she said the most important thing she wants is to have Jeremy out of the hands and control of certain people. Chris picked her up later that evening and she went home.

(*When Debra left, I came into the den and sobbed and sobbed until I couldn't breathe. Jerr came and comforted me and had tears in his eyes, too.*

Jerr: What do you think is going to happen, Lorr? What does Debra think is going to happen?

Lorr: I just don't know, sweetheart.

Jerr: Whatever it is, we told her we would be with her.

Lorr: This can't be happening, Jerr, this just can't be happening. What must she be thinking? What are her thoughts? I wish we could talk it out with her, but she's private about some things. I have to respect her feelings, no matter how it upsets us.)

12/10-18/09 —

Jerr and I spent the week shopping for Christmas presents — Old Navy, Best Buy, Sears, and Hallmark and then wrapping them with other gifts for the family. With us going to Florida for winters,

I have so much missed the Christmases we used to have. I mentioned this to Debra and she said, "Gee, Mom, what's a few years now when we had all those years with you for our Christmases and all the holidays. You have a life now and we have a different life. I'm not missing anything — well, maybe your 'Christmas Around the World' exhibit you used to put together. I always remember our house filled with Christmas music and you singing all the hymns and carols. Every room was decorated, even the bathrooms. I loved it. And don't forget, we chose to live elsewhere — Donna in Arizona and me in Depew and Niagara Falls. But we've always been together by phone and that's more personal in many ways. I could always feel a hug from you."

12/23/09, Wed., 2:30 P.M. —

Debra said she was finally feeling better (*however, I could hear her short of breath*); it seems like three or four days after her chemo treatment is when she feels really bad. She doesn't want to talk to or see anyone and doesn't go anywhere, then she bounces out of it for a week and then it's time for another treatment.

Upstate delivers Emend 125-80 mg.

Personal: Debra and Donna are going shopping tonight and thanked us for the gift cards. Debra had a long conversation yesterday with Phil; he was very upset about Debra's situation and didn't know what to say. She told him about the hysterectomy and the cervical cancer that was found, that she was referred to RPCI, had another major surgery and is receiving chemotherapy for stomach cancer. She needs his help now and he has to step up to the plate in helping with Jeremy, but it's like he just doesn't care. Jeremy was grounded, Phil took his cell phone, and computer and TV games away from him, then he very quietly sat him down and talked to him with no yelling. Debra's father said that this was his computer and he wants it back. He isn't getting it back. Phil and Debra agreed to stand together on this.

12/24/09, Thurs. —

Christmas gifts for Debra, Jeremy, and Donna. And gift certificates for Jeremy from Best Buy, Sears, Old Navy and Hallmark. Jeremy loves to shop for good clothes and always looks real nice. Debra is so proud of him. After the holidays, they enjoy shipping for bargains.

I went to Midnight Mass; prayed for the challenges in our entire family, in our friends' lives, and for Donna, Debra and Jeremy especially. I heard the beautiful music encircling our heads and hearts and thought how important faith was in our lives. How or from whom do people without faith accept such horrific news or walk through this valley without faith in our God, in our church, in our close community? This is more than the mind can comprehend. However, may they all find their own form of solace or faith. *Thank you, Jesus, for coming to earth.*

12/25/09, Fri. — Christmas Day.

It was a quiet day; we had cancelled our social visits and parties with friends. I was exhausted and just wanted to stay home. It was freezing cold.

12/28/09, Mon. —

Debra stayed with us overnight. We had our Christmas then, opened gifts, had munchies, laughed, but mostly were very quiet thinking of tomorrow. At one point, Debra and I were looking at the snow falling, and I told her, "Isn't it a miracle that no snowflake is like another one? That God created them to be so unique. I forget the molecular composition of just one snowflake which isn't important, only that He created all of us in the same way, each person is so unique. We have to thank Him for this miracle."

12/29/09, Tues. @ RPCI, Buffalo

Arose at 7:00 a.m., got us ready to leave for Debra's 8:00

appointment. It was freezing and the roads were slippery on the highways. We were a bit late. On our return home at 4:30 p.m., it was already dark and we hit the rush hour traffic after a long day, but we were doing what we needed to do and to support Debra. Our day was easy compared to hers.

12/29 - 30/09 - Chemo Procedure: Topotecan.

12/30/09, Wed. -Midnight — E/R at Millard Fillmore Suburban Hospital (MFSH) which is next door to us.

Debra is in severe pain. We've been there all night, she was given test after test, given an antibiotic prescription for an infection. She was finally discharged next day at 12:30 p.m.

We went to Perkins for lunch, then to a local store because Debra wanted reading glasses. She is having trouble with her eyes, and she laughed that she had to get "granny" glasses for the first time ever in her life! She told Jerr that next she was going to learn knitting, and he said, "Good, I'll get you one of those rocking chairs from the Cracker Barrel." She said, "Forget it, Jerr, they don't have them in black!" 🛴🛴 Chris picked her up later in the evening.

12/31/09, Thurs. —

"Happy New Year, Mom and Jerr. I love you two. And Jerrrry, to you, that *Felix* something or other." "*Feliz Ano Neuvo* — Happy New Year!" "*Debra, we pray that it will be a better year. We love you, sweetheart.*"

(*Prayer to St. Jude, the patron saint of the hopeless, for a full cure for Debra. As Catholics, we fall back on our source of appeals and know that prayer and petitions are the constancy of our religion. It is in prayer that we find solace and hope and peace. When you hit rock bottom, at least you know it's solid and solid enough to hold us when we reach up and out to God's love for us.*)

2010

THE CONTINUING TREATMENTS

Debra's changed schedule.

1/5-6-7/09 - Chemo Procedure: Topotecan.

1/5/10, Tues. —

Up at 8:00 a.m. — Another five hour treatment for Debra. She had some cold apple juice, the only beverage that would satisfy her. For lunch we bought her usual egg salad sandwich. Jerr sat in the rotunda and took a little snooze. The rotunda had a circular sofa with a tree growing in the middle and the walls were padded with a scenic mural, there was plush carpeting and soft music. I had read all the magazines the Clinic had on hand. I had forgotten my book and just sat and watched the patients come in and leave. Some of them looked hopeful and some had haunted-looking faces. Some wore old jogging suits and some were dressed smartly. We saw people with hats, caps, wigs, or with head gear at all. Some came alone and some were accompanied by a family member or friend. I said a prayer for all of them, both patient and whoever accompanied them. After Debra's five-hour treatment, we went to the Super Fuji Buffet for dinner. She was craving Chinese food!

1/6/10, Wed. —

Another five-hour treatment and the same routine. This time I had brought a book to read and was immersed in the riveting plot, when a woman flew out of the clinic sobbing in tears, ran across the atrium and punched the elevator button over and over again. I wanted to go and ask her if she was OK, but I knew she wasn't, and I wouldn't know what to say — maybe just hold her hand and cry. The elevator finally came, she entered the cab and I heard her punching the buttons. I put my book down, wiped a few tears and prayed, just prayed. And I asked why? Why?

We had dinner at IHOP at 5:00 p.m. Debra was not aware of the incident at the clinic and we didn't say anything. Upstate delivers Hydro/ACET.

1/7/10, Thurs. —

Today was Debra's last treatment for the week. We had a quick lunch at Tim Horton's on Transit as Debra's pain management doctor was back in the same building. This was the doctor who had been treating her for the 2005 car accident. The doctor gave Debra injections in her back and informed her that there was nothing more she could add to her pain meds than what she was being given by RPCI. The doctor was a lovely woman, so kind and caring and just sat and talked to us. I was happy we had finally met. I thanked her for her treatment of Debra — not only after she had been informed of Debra's diagnosis but years before that. She gave Debra a hug and clasped my hands. God bless her.

1/13/10, Wed. —

Debra was with us and we had a long talk about everything. We sat and talked about her treatments, the schedules, and the fact that her friend, Lisa and her husband, Doug, said that Lisa would be able to drive Debra to the Amherst Clinic for treatments. Many times, Lisa's mother had treatments on the same date but at another facility. It was bitter cold outside. We told her that she/ they could stay at our place overnight to make it easier to get to the

Amherst Clinic a mile away instead of coming from Niagara Falls 20 miles away. Debra said, "Mom, if anything happens, I am able to go to one of the hospitals for treatment from wherever I am. I have good medical care right now. I'm feeling better just a week after my treatments. I have Chris, I have Lisa and I'll be OK. *(But you don't have your mother and Jerr, sweetheart.)* Please don't delay your trip to Florida any longer, you usually leave in October or November. Jerr gets sick in the cold weather and I don't want to be responsible if he ends up in the hospital again. You know I can't visit him there!"

"Debra, we'll wait another week or so. We want to wait to see if you have a reaction from the chemo because that is usually when you react." (Don't *the chemo doctors know that? Can't they plan for that and assist their patients or do they just administer the chemo and hope nothing happens — or is Debra the only one getting these reactions? So many questions.* "Mom, please don't. I'll be all right."

Making the decision to depart for Florida, we again gave Debra and Donna all the food from the refrigerator and freezer and canned goods from the pantry.

Returning Debra home, we stopped for dinner at one of our favorite places — Como at the Airport. As usual, we were given over-sized entrees which added to more take-out packages we bought at their deli for Debra to take home. She went out loaded with bags, and we had to help her carry them to the car. Jerr pretended he was dragging the bags on the ground and we were laughing. "Come on, Jerr, toughen up those abs!", Debra called out. The aroma of Italian spices, spicy meatballs and sausages, the Como's spaghetti sauce and their special "pizza bread" coated with olive oil and herbs permeated the car, and we didn't want to open the doors — to not only let the icy cold wind into the warm car, but to not let Debra out! When we arrived at Chris' house, everyone helped carry the numerous bags. Hugs and kisses and hugs again and "we love you" over and over again. Driving home, the aroma was still in our car.

"Whew-ee, Jerr." We were laughing and Jerr said, "Well, sweetheart, that's our farewell gift!"

1/14/10, Thurs. —

We spent the day packing, making reservations at hotels along the way to Florida, got the car ready, went out for lunch, then dinner and to bed early. Several calls back and forth with Debra (*As usual, I couldn't sleep.*)

1/15/10, Fri. - 6:00 a.m. —

We set out for Florida — made the first stop at 3:30 p.m. — we were so tired. We called Debra several times during the day. She kept asking where we were. She said she was so worried until we got past the snow routes of Pennsylvania and the mountains and tunnels in West Virginia.

1/18/10, Mon. —

An early evening again. Four days later, we arrived in Florida, stopped for dinner, and then were greeted in the lobby by our best friend, Terri, and Mark who were waiting for us and then the rest of our family — the Library group! What fun, what a welcome, what friendship, what laughter!

We called Debra and she said she was OK.

1/22/10

Upstate delivers Emend 125-80 mg. to her.

1/24/10, Sun., 1:30 p.m. @ E/R NFMMH —

Debra has bronchitis again (*OH, NO!*) It took three hours to do a chest x-ray and blood work. Debra has been given two Z-pack antibiotics and will be given a prescription for the other two meds. She'll call us when she gets home, not to worry.

(*Jerr and I sat down and discussed returning to New York. He told me whatever I wanted to do, he would agree. No problem, but we're flying back.)*

Personal: Last week, Chris' son was in the hospital with the same bronchitis; he made them wear masks at the house. She thinks the older son also has it but he won't go to the hospital for treatment.

1/25/10, Mon. — Debra's call

She has finally been discharged from the E/R! We had four telephone conversations during the day. She's feeling better and will keep her appointment for chemo tomorrow. "I'm better, Mom, I really am."

Upstate delivers Emend 125-80 mg. to Debra.

1/26/10 - Chemo Procedure: Cisplatin

1/27/10

Upstate delivers Emend 125-80 mg.

1/27-28/10 - Chemo Procedure: Topotecan

Every day, several phone calls with Debra. Things are going OK.

2/15/10

Upstate delivers Emend 125-80 mg.

2/16/10, Tues. —

Donna is driving Debra to RPCI in Buffalo and then to the Amherst Clinic. On Wednesday and Thursday, Lisa will be taking Debra to Amherst. During Debra's January's treatment, Chris took the day off work to go with her. Debra took her pills and she was calm. Saturday to Saturday, she saw Dr. LaiLai and another practitioner, a Chinese person. There was heavy SNOW! Debra did not think she would make it to her treatments.

2/18, 19, 20/10 - Chemo Procedure: ?

2/19/10, Wed. — Upstate delivers Lorazepam*, 1 mg.

2/25/10, Thurs. —

Debra was so happy; she went to Bon Ton's big sale and for $30 bought Jeremy's shorts and shirts for the Florida trip, as he had outgrown his clothes from last year. He can probably wear the same shorts but needs tan sandals in size 10-12. She's feeling good; next week she'll probably go back and look for something for herself. She's going to buy a wig at a shop she saw. Laughing, she didn't know if she was going to be a blond, redhead or brunette!

👍 👍 (*It doesn't matter, sweetheart, we'll know it's YOU!*)

Debra is very tired; she's worried about Jeremy; it's 45 degrees outside and very cold. CT scan scheduled for 3/30. "Mom, I did not file a tax return — had no income. How many years have I ever missed filing a tax return — never since I started working! It makes me feel terrible. It makes me feel useless. What if the IRS comes after me?"

3/8/10, Mon. — Donna's call

She had been in the hospital since Wednesday, 3/3/10. (*OMG, now what?!*) She had very severe chest pain and numbness in her left hand; they asked her if she pulled her muscles or hurt her neck. Debra took her to the E/R, and she was later admitted; put on a heart monitor; given an EKG; extensive blood work done; her enzymes were very low. Good news — she does not have high cholesterol! She was given nitro, but she threw it up and it gave her a severe headache. Deb stayed with Donna's two dogs at her apartment from 10:00 a.m. to 5:30 p.m. Doctors determined that Donna had a cardiac condition and was told to follow-up with her doctor on Monday. She was instructed to continue Crestor, morphine, Zanax. Until she gets the endometriosis* treated, the tumors will push on her stomach and she becomes ill to her stomach. She has suffered with this condition for years.

In the midst of all this, Donna will take Debra for her 5-hour treatment. (*Donna's dogs are a special breed called Basenji. They are African hunting dogs but are the dogs depicted to be guarding the Egyptian pyramids. They are known as the "barkless dog," but when excited, they make a noise that sounds like a little yodel. Their colors include chestnut red, pure black or brindle -- all with white feet, chest and tail tip. They also don't shed their fur. Their tails curl into a circle. Really smart, beautiful dogs.*)

3/10/10 - CT scan performed.

3/10/10 —

After a gut-wrenching decision, Debra had finally resigned herself to getting a wig for when she comes to Florida. When Debra and Donna stopped at the RPCI Wig Center (located behind the cafeteria), someone yelled at them "You can't come in here; I'm busy helping this lady!" All this woman saw were two young-looking girls trying to enter her realm, she did not see a cancer patient who had reached a heartbreaking decision and needed compassion! Later, Debra was crying and saying "OMG, Mom, OMG, when was the last time anybody spoke to me like that?"

3/15/10

Upstate delivers Emend 125-80 mg.

3/24/10 - CT Scan performed.

4/5/10, Mon. —

"Mom, I will go to my appointment on Tuesday. My feet hurt and my toe nails are so long."

Personal: Jeremy has a new computer password, and it is locked up. Debra called Chris who said he could not unlock the computer. We had to drive Jeremy home and he took the laptop with him. Phil grounded Jeremy. Her father said he had to go to the VA hospital; he was screaming and yelling; so miserable.

At Donna's work, a lady fell in the lobby and was bleeding so Donna took her to the hospital and waited with her all night until 1:00 a.m.

"Mom, there is so much chaos here, I'm stressed with everybody's problems, — on and on and on!"

Debra, I understand you are in the midst of all these problems, but you know that stress and anger is not good for you. Let's try to see the positive side of ....

"Mom, you have no idea what is happening around here — it's disappointing. It's what I have to live with — yes, all around me! Bye!" Hanging up.

11:00 p.m. (sobbing) "Mom, I'm so sorry for snapping at you. I love you and I know you have our best interests at heart. You have always tried to solve things and calm things down and get people together. Sometimes I don't think that is possible in this family! People have too many agendas and they won't change. Nothing changes — ever! You have your faith and the rest of us just have.... LIFE!!! 🛇 🛇

Debra, I love you, too, sweetheart. You are going through so much, I don't know how you do it. I always thought you were the fragile one, my Princess, and the courage I've seen in how you handle this situation. I don't know how you do it, really. I don't even know how I would cope. I only pray that you will come through this.

Mom, I'm not courageous; I'm scared, and it hurts and it's so foreign, but your calm ways and Jerry's "let's do it, kiddo" attitude — just keeps me taking one step after the other. I distract myself with TV or magazines. I try not to even think about it.

4/6/10, Tues. @ RPCI for chemo.

Debra's crying over her hair loss. She never removes her cap. "Mom, all my hair has fallen out; it's nothing but peach fuzz growing behind my ears and neck about three inches long. My scalp hurts — feels like it has a burn."

On Tuesday when Donna took Debra to RPCI, her father called Donna and asked her to come home now and start the computer for him. Donna said she couldn't because Jeremy had changed all the passwords. Later, Debra told me, she was crying her eyes out about all the problems and was taking gulping gasps.

Personal: *"Why didn't anyone call us when Donna was in hospital?"* Later, we were told she didn't want anyone to know she wasn't eating properly and that is what made her ill.

Debra has to apply for Social Security Disability; she was so desperate (she got food stamps to help Chris with bills; she eats chicken, beef, veggies, milk.) "Mom, why do I have to do this degrading stuff? I want to be able to stand on my own two feet again. I hate depending on anybody!"

Personal: "Mom, Jeremy has shot up to 6'2" and weighs 200 lbs. and is all muscle from working out. He can hardly wait to get to Florida and has saved his money to buy a T-shirt at the Hard Rock!"

4/13/10, Tues. - 11:00 p.m. Debra's call

She didn't get a chance to talk to me today. She was at Lisa's house; told her the good news. (*What good news, sweetheart?*) Dr. LaiLai's assistant, the Indian woman, was the one who called her with the "Good News". The CT scan revealed the cancer was all gone, except a tiny spot left; it's so small they can't even measure it; the five BIG SPOTS ARE GONE! (*Praise the Lord!*) Debra's white platelets are down; they will go down after the chemo, but she has the ability to get them right back up.

Lisa made dinner; they had a wine cooler. Lisa: "Debra, it must be the way you're acting; your hair knew you loved it so much, you weren't going to lose it." The doctors want to do one more chemo treatment when she gets back to Buffalo from Florida. There's also one tiny spot on her lungs which they said they are not concerned about, but they want everything GONE! They will probably tell her they are going to monitor her in the future. She eats a lot of protein, steaks, broccoli, cauliflower, vitamin water, etc.

I called RPCI about the 3/9/10 incident when Debra and Donna went into the Wig Center. I was connected to the Breast Resource/Community Resource Center for the Wig Center. I spoke to a Karen, then a Jo-Ann, and finally Diana, who informed me she is at the Wig Center Monday through Friday but was probably off on 3/9/10. Diana told me she can custom-order a wig with long hair; she will help Debra personally. "Mom, forget it. I'll never go in there again!"

4/19/10 to 4/25/10, Mon.-Sun. —

Deb and Jeremy arrive in Florida on Jet Blue for a 6-day visit!

4/19/10, Mon. —

Stopped at Giorgio's Bistro for breakfast. Jeremy loved the location right on the Intracoastal — a big change from Buffalo weather.

4/20/12, Tues. —

Spent the day at the pool with naps on the chaise lounges. We then went for dinner at Cadillac Ranch in Gulfstream Village and sat outside on the patio under umbrellas. Afterward, we stopped at Party City and bought an insulated mini-cooler for the plane trip home. The two of them said they did not want to buy any airport food! Then a stop at a grocery store for mini-juice cans and nibbles. We packed our own sandwiches, fruit and cookies (even though we now know it wasn't the food at the New York Airport which caused Debra's problems last year.)

4/21/10, Wed, —

Deb purchased Nerf football for Jeremy at a drugstore and bought his favorite milk — regular milk. (*We drink 2%, skim, or lactose-free milk.*) We spent the day at the ocean and had lunch at Rocco's Pizza — Jeremy's request. Then bought Debra some white tank tops because it was really warm! Arrived back home for a short rest at the pool and then that evening went to the Hard Rock Café for dinner. We bought Debra her sparkly Hard Rock Hollywood T-shirt. Jeremy had saved money to get his own. In the evening, we went to the pool again and the two of them went swimming. We sat under the canopy or along the Intracoastal and talked quietly for hours. It was a beautiful day and evening,

4/22/10, Thurs, —

We went on the Jungle Queen Cruise boat again — this was a must. Does it change? No, but it's "tradition" and both of them are comforted by things we always do together. Then we stopped at the Nexxt Café in Miami for dinner.

4/23/10, Thurs. —

Another trip to Aventura Mall where we bought Ghirardelli Chocolates for their trip home -- with Jerr sneaking some for his secret stash! We were laughing — as if I didn't know he had the "stash"! 🔒 🔒

4/24/10, Sat. —

We got up early and went for breakfast at Giorgio's Bistro and then spent a lazy day around the pool, having lunch under the turquoise canopy. That evening we went to China Canton for dinner.

4/25/10, Sun. —

Up really early for their flight back home. Stopped for breakfast at.......yup, you guessed it — at McDonald's! Jeremy told his mom,

"Mom, we just have to do the 'usual things'." Once again, off they flew, and we sadly returned home. We told them we had decided to leave Florida within the next three weeks.

4/26/10, Mon. —

Upstate delivers Emend 125-80 mg. Dexamethasone 4 mg.

4/27/10 - Tues. — Debra's call

She is being given yet another kind of shot. *(For what?)* She doesn't know. Apparently, she isn't going to be discharged today. Her words were slurry but not as bad as when I spoke to her on Friday. All she does is sleep. They were giving her Xanex but now are giving her Zoloft for depression. *(Why?)* So many questions and no answers.

Upstate delivers Lorazepam 1 mg.

4/27, 28, 29/10 - Chemo procedure.

4/30/10, Fri. - 1:00 p.m. @ RPCI Amherst Clinic —

Debra has finished her chemo treatment. The nurses had a lot of trouble with the needles. They couldn't get into the veins in her hands even though she drank a lot of water; her hands are black and blue. She told the nurses that her body was ejecting the treatment because it wasn't needed. ⚓⚓ They said "Probably so". The nurse on Thursday tried twice and then another nurse got a different needle and tried twice. They gave her Xanex; she felt very tired all week, but today feels good. She will continue with the last treatment in May and then have the CT scan and hopefully the "good news."

5/8/10, Sun. Mother's Day — Debra's call

Early morning — "Happy Mother's Day, Mummy!" "Happy Mother's Day to you, sweetheart. Thank you for your beautiful card."

"Mom, I meant every word. Hallmark seems to know what I wanted to say and they wrote it for me!" 🕯️🕯️ Our card to Debra was just as special and loving. Jeremy had given her a beautiful card, and she just loved it. She said she held it to her breast and just smiled.

Donna's card said: I was going to surprise you on MOTHER'S DAY, Mom!!! But I figured having me was enough of a surprise for one lifetime! Happy Mother's Day! Love always, Donna

I love my girls! We agreed to celebrate Mother's Day when we returned from Florida. The date doesn't matter, the love does and it will be there on any date.

5/16/10, Sun. — En route to New York

Early morning, Jerr and I left Florida — driving only five or six hours each day and stopping at our usual favorite places — Vero Beach, St. Augustine, Mile Marker 29 in Georgia (thanks to friends, Bill and Jo-Ann who introduced us to the Rah Bar), Charleston, South Carolina, North Carolina, then in West Virginia at Tamarack, then the New River Gorge scenic overlook. Driving through the two tunnels, and reaching Pennsylvania, we know that we're only six hours away. We stop at our usual place for lunch in Grove City, PA — "Eat 'N Park" where we buy their famous SMILE cookies for the kids and friends. We walk off our lunch by strolling through all the outlet stores and proceed on our trip, finally we encounter the "Stop at toll booth" sign — the first toll we've been subjected to in 2,200 miles. Welcome to New York State!

5/18/10

Upstate delivers Emend 125-80 mg, Effexor* XR 75 mg.

5/18, 19, 20/10 - Chemo Procedure: Topotecan.

5/18/10, Tues. —

Debra had her 5-hour treatment today; the nurses had a lot of trouble with the needles. Debra had not been feeling well since last week but didn't want to tell us. Chris was at home sick with flu; then his son came down with it; then Debra did. She thinks it's a 48-hour thing, but she told the nurse about it when she went in.

5/19/10, Wed. —

We arrived back in New York. We bypass the second toll booth a few miles further and exit at Main Street in Williamsville, taking the side roads. We stopped at the first Tim Horton's on Main for a snack dinner — now we know we're back.

Debra had said she was scheduled for a chemo treatment on 5/18/10 and we anxious to see her and talk to her. Then calls to Donna and Jeremy and to friends back in Florida that we had arrived safely.

5/19/10, Wed. —

During Debra's chemo treatment, the nurses again had a lot of trouble with the needles; they couldn't get them in. I could see Debra becoming agitated, and she gave me that "I want to leave" look. I sat by her but could not watch. Tom, one of the male nurses, came over and said, "Use a smaller needle." The nurse told Tom that with the larger needle, the chemo goes in faster. He replied, "With the smaller one, yes, it will take longer." He went back to his own patient. (*It takes longer? Well, so what? For whose convenience is that?! I was furious! After all this time?!*)

We picked Debra up and she stayed with us overnight. (*I sat and cried at the pain she was experiencing, and I couldn't do anything about it to help.*)

5/20/10, Thurs. —

The schedule was the same, she had her 5-hour treatment, we had lunch and when she was finished, we came home. Debra was not feeling well and was very tired. Chris drove over in the evening and picked her up.

5/21/10, Fri., 8:00 p.m. @ NFMMH —

Debra called and told us that during the night, she was so sick and finally in the morning, she went to the E/R with severe muscle pains in her upper thighs, in her arms, and she had trouble breathing. She was admitted; had a CT scan and she was told there were spots on her lungs, and they were inflamed. (*What?*) She called RPCI in Amherst; spoke to Reney, who called Dr. LaiLai. She is being given pain medication, it was found that her blood sugar was very high, and the doctors began giving her meds for that (*insulin?*), and Heparin. (*What is this for?*) (*Jerr's brother, Mark said Heparin was for the prevention of blood clots.*)

Debra is getting shots in the stomach, and she is black and blue. She heard that she would be discharged.

Debra told us that if she had had this kind of reaction to the chemo after her first treatment, she would never have continued with the treatments. She would have taken what would come. But then she said, "Mom, I think it's a way of showing me compassion for those people who cry and are very depressed about their treatments." She could never understand them; she thought she could talk herself out of it. YOU CAN'T! Before she continues with any more chemo, she said, "They are going to have to show me proof that I need them!" She's scheduled again in June but says, "NO, not right now I don't want them!"

She saw another pain doctor at the hospital, who took 9,000 tests, every time he gives her something, Heparin, shot causes high blood sugar, CT Scan, nodule on lung, inflamed, did call Dr. LaiLai;

pain from bladder infection? She's nauseous and has head-to-toe pain; it hurts. She was fatigued, couldn't climb stairs, very weak, muscles hurt, constantly in pain, arms, back, legs, side effects, she's winded, has a pain shot every 2 hours; half a treatment, not on oxygen. Her words are slurred.

During her chemo treatments this week, the first needle went in OK; the second one, she sat up on the couch, but the third one — cried when they were trying to push in needle in again. Finally, Tom came over and again said to use the smaller needle. (*Wouldn't that have been in her record?!*)

While Debra was in the hospital, Dr. LaiLai (Renee) said don't worry about missing the last chemo treatment; you have no virus. Her sugar level had came down from the original high recording. She's being given pain meds. every three hours; she can feel it wear off in about 2-½ hours because her muscles start to cramp up. Sodium chloride - 3 EKG, fine, glands under her jaw are swollen.

5/22/10, Sat. @ NFMMH — Debra's call

She is being given yet another kind of shot, for what she doesn't know. Apparently, she isn't going to be discharged today. Her words were slurry but not as bad as when I spoke to her on Friday. All she does is sleep. They were giving her Xanex but now are giving her Zoloft for depression. (*Why?*) So many questions and no answers. When we went to see her, she was still sleepy.

5/23/10, Sun. @ NFMMH —

Went to see Debra after St. Gregory Church services. I stopped at the Grotto to say prayers for my daughter. I feel so hopeless and out of control. I feel I have to put her in God's hands because some days, I can't even say the name of Jesus or our familiar prayers. She was feeling better but not 100% she said.

5/24/10, Mon. — Debra's call

She was being discharged and for us not to come to the hospital as she has a ride home. She'll call us later this evening.

5/24/10 to 6/15/10 —

We've had twenty-two days without problems. (*Praise, God, and thank You.*)

6/14/10, Mon. —

Debra stayed overnight with us. On our way back, we stopped at Wegmans and she bought all her favorite foods to take home later. he has already had dinner today — what little she could eat — and didn't want to eat with us — except ICE CREAM BARS, yummy 🍦🍦, she said. She said she's hungry but the sight or smell of food makes her feel nauseated. She was very nervous about tomorrow.

Upstate delivers Emend 125-80 mg.

6/15, 16, 17/10 - Chemo Procedure: Topotecan.

6/15/10, Tues. — @ RPCI Amherst Clinic

Her 5-hour chemo treatment and again problems with the needles.

We had lunch at Perkin's after her treatment.

6/16/10, Wed. —

Upstate Pharmacy delivered Oxycodone 10 mg for Debra.

6/16/10, Wed. —

Debra wanted an egg salad sandwich at the Grateful Deli; she loves them. She was tired and slept all afternoon during her treatment. We had dinner at home.

6/17/12, Thurs. —

After Debra's chemo, we stopped at Anderson's in Williamsville — Jerr and Debra wanted their rare roast beef sandwiches, and of course their scrumptious ice cream. (*My choice is always the grilled chicken sandwich.*) Chris picked Debra up and she went home.

Nineteen days without problems. (*Please God, let her be healed, in Your infinite mercy, You can heal her.*)

6/28/10, Mon. —

"Happy birthday, sweetheart." "Thank you, Mom." She loved her birthday card and Jerr's message on it. We were laughing. We had made arrangements to celebrate her birthday next week.

Upstate delivers Effexor XR 75 mg.

7/1/10, Thurs. —

We celebrate Debra's birthday with "lundin" at Orazio's in Clarence. She and Jerr ordered steak and I had my usual salmon. Chris met her after work and she went home.

That evening, we took Jeremy to Bison Baseball field for "Drums Along the Waterfront". An exciting, dynamic performance and competition. We rode the Metrorail to and from the field; it departs from the University station by our home and there's a stop directly in front of the field. We ate our fill of food and drinks.

7/2/10, Fri. —

Today we shopped at Marshall's and Macy's for Debra's present, and she chose comfortable, summer clothes.

7/7/10, Wed. — CT scan of chest/abdomen/pelvis.

After her test, we had "lundin" at the Olive Garden.

7/9/10, Fri. —

Jerr had a doctor's appointment and Debra wanted to come with us. "It's about time that I'm on the other side of the bed, Jerr!" We stopped for lunch at the Sheridan Family Restaurant for pitas and Greek salads and soup.

7/10/10, Sat. —

We arose early and went to Coffee Culture in Williamsville for breakfast and then down to Farmer's Market where we strolled around, listened to the wonderful music by live musicians, smelled and bought the freshly baked bread and rolls, the freshly ground coffee beans, the tangy cheese, the smooth wine samples, selecting fresh vegetables and fruits. We even purchased jars of jam from "Mother" — an elderly lady with a wonderful, beaming smile. She dresses in a frilly white cap and apron and a printed dress. She bottles her own jams and jellies and has her photo on the jars. Debra selected a bouquet of flowers for the dining room.

7/13/10 - Scheduled Chemo cancelled after blood work and check-up.

7/13/10, Tues. —

Up at 8:00 for breakfast and the drive to Buffalo. Debra's blood results were not good enough; chemo has been postponed. ♀ "Bummer", she said. However, during the hour wait, we were at the GYN clinic on the 2nd floor, and we were listening to the piano music drifting up through the atrium. It was beautiful and all of a sudden, Debra is crying and then bends over and starts sobbing. Jerr and I looked at each other? When she finally got a hold of herself, I was holding her hand and asked, "Debra, sweetheart, are you in pain? What can I do?" "Oh, Mummy, I was just remember-ing the way you used to play the piano with the same music we are hearing. And you would sing and sing and sing. I would love "Amazing Grace" the best because you sang it with such feeling.

I understand every word now." Other patients were looking at us and one woman offered up her appointment time so Debra could be taken sooner. She told the kind woman that she wasn't going to be seen by the doctor, and that we were just awaiting the results of the blood test. "Oh, Mom, what a gift some people are."

When Debra had the results and was informed that she wasn't going to be treated, she said, "Let's stop at the Anchor Bar again for lunch, Jerrrrry?" At lunch, Debra had a turkey club, but she kept putting her nose up and smelling the spicy Buffalo chicken wings and sauce on our plates. She was smiling, "Oh, boy, do I miss those, but they would ruin my stomach." After lunch, we dropped Debra off at our home and went to Dash's and bought balloons for her — ones that said "Princess" (which has been my nickname for her since she was a little girl! She was like the Princess in the fable of "The Princess and the Pea." She laughed every time I called her that.) 🛁🛁

Upstate delivers Emend 125-80 mg, Dexamethasone 4 mg.

7/14/10, Wed. —

We continued shopping at Kohl's near our house for more clothes for Debra.

7/16/10, Fri. —

Went to the drugstore to get Debra's prescription for pain meds. She couldn't wait for the next day's delivery when she got home.

7/23/10, Tues. — Chemo Procedure.

7/26/10, Mon. —

Upstate Pharmacy called us in Williamsville to confirm delivery of Debra's prescription for Effexor (for depression) and Acetaminophen. We told him to call her in Niagara Falls, she was back home. I hang up and am wondering again about the "depression" statement. I suppose anyone facing chemo treatments are going to be depressed. Debra has never mentioned it.

Upstate delivers Emend 125-80 mg.

7/28/10, Wed. —

Debra feels much better; there's no humidity. Tried calling the RPCI nurse, voice mail after voice mail; left message; coming over on Tuesday as usual.

"Mom, listen to this. I wanted a prescription refill for pain meds from the pain management doctor. The pharmacist said it had expired and that a new one was needed every month now. I called the doctor's office in Amherst, and the girl was so nasty and said, 'After all this time you've been coming into the office and you didn't know this?' " Debra was crying. She said the medicine had recently been changed, and no one said anything about this now being a month-to-month refill, instead of a 90 day supply. After being put on hold for 15 minutes, the office clerk said they would make an exception this time because on this kind of medicine, the request has to be placed seven days prior to the expiration date and then it's mailed to pharmacy.

7/20/10, Fri. —

Chris is off work and will drive Debra to the Amherst doctor's office to pick the prescription up in person. She sees that doctor again in October. Their voice message informs patients to place refill orders only, no other information. Chris then took Debra to the Park Avenue Coat Company to get her the jacket she wanted for her birthday.

8/5/10 - Chemo Procedure: CPK Chemo Taxol/Carbo

8/6/10 - No chemo.

8/5/10, Thurs. - 8:00 a.m. —

Debra had discussed with us that she does not want to continue with this protocol. (*Please, God, let us make the right decision.*) She would tell Dr. LaiLai when she goes for blood work and the usual internal exam at Amherst. She told him she does not want to continue with this protocol. What are the ramifications of stopping treatment for a while, then having a CT scan to see where she is? Dr. LaiLai apparently told her he could use another form of chemo with not as serious side effects. *(Really? After all this time?!)*

Jerr had a scheduled doctor's appointment, and we left to keep that appointment as it was only a couple blocks away. Debra had said she would wait for us downstairs in the atrium. That is what we expected when we returned. She wasn't there. We parked and went upstairs to the clinic. The nurses had already started the different treatment! I asked her, "What happened?" She just shook her shoulders and looked at us with that look that she didn't want to discuss it right now. No privacy.

By the time we got home, she was crying and crying. "Why is he doing this to me, Mummy? Doesn't he listen to me? Doesn't anyone listen to me?! I told him I didn't want to continue and when he told me about the different chemo, I thought it would be started next time. I wanted more information and then I would make my own decision. All of a sudden, a nurse came and got me and started the IV! What was I going to say in front of everybody — because there's no privacy, and you know everybody's business, fight with her? I think they were angry because I wasn't on their precious schedule. I feel the nurses and staff were talking about me."

(All I could do was hold her and hold her and cry with her. I was so angry I didn't know what to do. I wanted to go there and rip the place apart [not really] but was so angry.) Then I told her, *Don't worry about what people say behind your back. They are the people who are finding faults in your life instead of fixing the faults in their own life. Can you imagine*

working in such a place every day, all day long and then being at the
mercy of a doctor who does and says what he wants. It wasn't you, it was
them and the doctor. Forget them, Debra." "Mom, it just feels like "get
'em in, get 'em out, goodbye."

We had ice cream bars at home and Debra went to bed early. She
said she was dreading the next day.

8/6/10, Fri., 7:30 a.m. —

Debra woke up with severe pain in her spine, her feet were numb
and her hands were starting to get numb. By 8:00 a.m., she needed
to go to the hospital immediately for IV pain meds. Millard
Fillmore is next door and while she was attended to immediately,
she did not get relief until 2:00 p.m., crying with the severe pain.
She got three doses and finally the third one worked.

Debra was discharged twelve hours later, with a prescription for
Lortab 10 mg, to continue with ibuprofen (Motrin) 600 mg, four
times a day for pain, venlafaxine* (Effexor XR), 75 mg, every day.
Stop taking Oxycodone 10 mg-acetaminophen (Percocet 7.5/325).
We went to the drug store, and they filled it. By the time we took
her home, she was non-stop talking, happy, and relief from pain.
"Mom, I say again that in my whole life I never even had to take an
aspirin and now this? What's happening to me? "

Also, on the drive home, our usual classical station was softly
playing. The *Ave Maria* came on, and I started singing it, then Jerr
joined in, and we were both singing the beautiful words. I could
see Debra in the back seat listening, then put her head down for a
moment, with tears. When the notes drifted away, Jerr and I looked
at each other, and he reached for my hand and gently squeezed it.
Debra quietly said, "That was beautiful to hear both of you singing
— especially you Jerr!" *(Yes, BOTH of us singing!)*

Cuba: Debra had heard Jerr's story as a little Jewish boy growing
up in Cuba, wandering around the neighborhoods. He would do

his little tasks all week. and one Friday when he was walking home, he heard beautiful music coming from a Catholic church and saw all the little boys going in. So he went in to see what was going on. After a while, he kept going in every time he saw the boys going in to sing. It turned out that the boys were a choir and he joined them. He went for months until one day his mother found out and — OH BOY! But I always said that with the right training, Jerr could have been a professional tenor — although he said he wanted to be a doctor or attorney! The poverty and hunger, even before Castro, was rampant, and the boys tried their hands at any little task or job that would give them a couple of pennies or a nickel to bring home to their mother. That's why when a charismatic Castro gave his inspirational speeches and promised the people everything, they believed him until he became their dictator and slowly, methodically, he took everything away from the people.

8/9/10, Mon. —

I sent Sharon Debra's FAX again asking for Lab reports and the CT Scan record. (*Never received them.*)

8/10/10, Tues. — Pain Management Clinic — Dr. Abraham.

After Debra's appointment, we stopped at Spot Coffee.

8/17/10, Tues. — Chemo Procedure: Taxotere/Carboplatin.

Debra was given a Patient Results print-out for her blood test that day. After her chemo, she had an appointment in the same building at her pain management doctor who gave her shots in her back. Then we stopped at Bagel Jay's for late lunch.

8/26/10

Upstate delivers Emend 125-80 mg.

8/25, 26, 27/10 - Chemo Procedure: Adriamycin*, CPK Chemo CTX/Adria*.

8/26/10, Thurs . —

Had "lundin" at the Cracker Barrel after her chemo. She hadn't felt like having lunch today but by the time she was finished, she was famished.

8/27/10, Fri. —

Tonight we had dinner at Perkins. Chris picked her up later that evening.

9/3/10, Fri. —

Debra is experiencing severe pain in her upper breastbone; nothing alleviates it. Does she need to go to the hospital? She said she would wait a while, she doesn't want to go. She will try to sleep but it's terrible.

9/4/10, Sat., 1:00 a.m. @ E/R NFMMH

She was admitted after five hours. They will contact Dr. LaiLai and are running tests. My friend in Florida, Linda, called and suggested that perhaps it was a gallbladder attack which was severely painful. She and other friends had it and that's what it is. (*If that's what it is, thank God, the doctors can fix it.*) Debra had mentioned it to the doctors; they want to do a scope but have to clear it with Dr. LaiLai first.

When she arrived in the E/R, the doctor and the nurses she liked were there; they said her platelets are very low; she was crying; writhing on the floor with the pain. Two young Indian doctors came in, then interns came in; it's not an ulcer and not in her lung (she would be having difficulty breathing, they said). She hasn't eaten for three days so it's not heartburn; her bowel movements (b/m) are OK.

Personal: We talked about Donna's situation.

9/8/10, Wed. @ NFMMH —

Debra will be started on blood transfusions of A positive blood as they can't get her platelets up. She feels like a pin cushion; the tips of her fingers are so sore; they come and take blood every hour it seems. (*Both Jerr and I have wished we could donate blood for her or in her name, but we can't. I thank everybody who can donate blood for people like my daughter. May God bless you.*)

We talked to her later and she will be given four bags of blood. At 8:00 p.m., she was on her third bag. She has finally been eating; the dietician discussed her diet, and it was her usual diet — turkey, fruit. The dietician was surprised that Debra had no complaints about the food, saying as she smiled at her, " I love the food."

9/9/10, Thurs. @ NFMMH —

Talked to Debra several times. She will be given several tests today and for us not to come to the hospital yet.

9/10/10, Fri. @ NFMMH —

Debra was given an upper GI series, a lower GI series, her spleen is fine, her heart is fine, and her lungs are fine. Tomorrow morning she should get the final results of these two tests. The only test they could not do is the scope of her heart although Dr. LaiLai told her the chemo that she just had will affect her heart. (*What?*) And it's not gallbladder! She feels like she has an ulcer; she has pain in the middle of her back, on left ribs, and between her breastbones. "It feels like I have the flu," she says. She was given a pain patch and a Sentinel pain shot. She wants to see all the test results.

Personal: Her father kept calling Donna because he didn't know why Debra was transferred to ICU; he came to the hospital tonight with Jeremy. She had her hat on so Jeremy didn't say anything about her hair. She didn't have her phone in ICU so Chris brought her phone charger and we can now contact her.

9/11/10, Sat. @ NFMMH —

The oncologist asked Debra, "What are you being treated for at RPCI?" She said, "Stomach cancer." He responded, "Well, Debra, from your CT scan, **we see no evidence of it!**"

Then Dr. Kondroskova (This *doctor is the one who found her ulcer last year*) rushed into Debra's room, telling the nurses to disconnect all the IV pain meds they were pumping in her. The doctor told Debra, "My little chickadee, we have found you have shingles* and we will treat you for them immediately!" None of the pain meds would touch the shingles! The doctor started giving her on a tiny white pill for the shingles plus other pills. Within twenty-five minutes, she was finally free from this pain. She's very sleepy. Later, the doctors said it was because Debra did not break out in blisters on the surface of her skin that it mislead them. All the blisters were on the inside, and yes, it causes severe pain! "Oh, gosh, Mom, what a blessing this doctor is. I thank God for her. I had the feeling that everybody here thought I was faking about the pain or that I was crazy." (*Much later, I researched shingles and one of the causes is CHEMOTHERAPY! Wouldn't this have been a path that Dr. LaiLai would have considered?*)

9/12/10, Sun. @ NFMMH —

A nurse came in and gave Debra the 1-½ hour "spa treatment". She was laughing because it was so personal, but she was washed from head to foot, her feet soaked in warm water; the bedding and her clothing changed. She was given another pint of blood, her white cells are still low — four points down. When she was admitted, she was almost down to 1! She was told, "We almost lost you, Debra." Oral pain med for **shingles**, her skin is sensitive, she has mid-back pain. She's being given a pain patch which won't make her break out. She was informed that anybody who has had chicken pox can get shingles. Everyone needs to wear gloves/masks/ gowns to prevent infection, and Debra needs bottled water NOT tap water.

She told the nurse that now she feels like she has a cold and a headache. The nurse said it is from the oxygen. During the night, she was given four more blood transfusions. When Jerr and I left the hospital, we were so exhausted; we stopped at the Como at the Airport Restaurant for dinner.

9/14/10, Tues. — RPCI Pain Clinic appointment.

9/14/10, Tues. —

Finally, the day arrived when she would meet with the RPCI pain management doctor. She craved for this meeting and opportunity to discuss her condition. A treatment would be prescribed, and she will have relief. The first thing the doctor stated was that her back pain was from her car accident (*Five years ago?*) Debra told him, "No, it's not; I know what that pain felt like then and have been treated for it. This is much more severe and in a different area. It goes from the middle of my breastbone to my back. It's not from the accident!" The doctor told her, "You don't know." Debra said. "Yes, I do know! It's been my body, and I know everything about it now, and if you aren't going to help me, then this place is useless to me."

She walked out and called me on my cell phone, as we were sitting in the lobby listening to the beautiful music. She was shaking, sobbing and almost ran out of the hospital, didn't want to speak to anybody. People were staring at us. In the car, she continued crying, "Why don't they believe me, Mom? I know what I'm talking about! I thought finally this place would help me and they didn't! They didn't!" (*The 2005 X-rays and subsequent ones show that her back injury was in the neck and lower back! She was complaining about pain in her breastbone and upper back. Did RPCI have these records? Did they request these X-rays from the treating doctor or from Debra? When her back treatment was completed, she was given the X-rays. No, the doctors didn't listen to her, just made an off-the-cuff assumption.*)

Debra asked me to call RPCI as she was too upset. I spoke to Charron and related the information that Debra never wanted to return to their Pain Clinic and did Debra have to keep her chemo appointment on Thursday? "No," Charron said. Debra requested that all the labs and the CT scan be faxed to her and that she was cancelling all her chemo treatments for now until she saw Dr. LaiLai. Charron said in a monotone to "give her a big hug from me". (*Yeah, right!*)

9/15/10, Wed. — @ NFMMH

At about midnight, Debra had to go to the E/R. During the night, she was transferred from the E/R to CCU on the 3rd Floor. Later, her regular doctor came in and said everything was fine; she was going to release her on Thursday and send her home with prescriptions.

9/16/10, Thurs. —

Upstate delivers Hydromorphone 2 mg, Effexor XR 75 mg.

9/16/10, Thurs. — Chemo Procedure: Cisplatin.

Debra's not feeling well today; she's real tired; feels like she has a cold or the flu; during the night her temperature rose to 100°. Doctor asked if she wanted to go home and she told him, "Yes, but not until I feel better, because I do not want to come back in a few days, and go through this all over again." She is sleeping, feels OK, another chest X-ray was done. Her throat hurts but her temperature is down. An Oriental doctor came in, didn't say anything, looked, then turned around and left. "What am I, an exhibit?" She's still on antibiotics plus eight other meds. Doctors are doing blood cultures (organism) for two days; nurses have no more places left to take blood, they had to take it from inside the wrist which really HURT! "Mommy, why? Why?"

9/19/10, Sun. — Debra is really weak this time. She's so, so tired and has flashes of nausea.

Personal: Debra was going to spend the day with us when Chris called her. His mother called and said her husband, Tom, had died and Chris was on his way to Lewiston. Ginny had to go into work for two customers (she's a hair dresser). Tom had asked her not to go to work but then he always said that. When she returned at 11:15 a.m. - 1-½ hours later — he had passed away.

9/19/10, Sun. —

My usual trek to St. Gregory's and prayers for Debra and our extended families and all their joys, problems, and challenges.

Debra is feeling much better. (*Thank God.*) She worked on Lisa's garden, as she had promised her at beginning of summer. Jeremy came over on Saturday and played with Lisa's son in the back yard but kept coming over every half-hour to ask, "Mommy, does your back hurt?" She said "No! Not at all." He couldn't believe it; he was so happy and was smiling for the first time in a long time. Debra had spent most of the summer in bed and in pain. Lisa has also had a bad back but kept trying to help Debra. After they were finished with the garden, Deb and Jeremy went for a walk in their woods and he asked her why she had lost her hair. Deb said, "The medicine that they are giving me will make you lose your hair." He asked, 'How long are you going to be sick?' Deb responded, "Hopefully, only one more month, honey."

9/20/10, Mon. —

"Mummy, I HAVE NO PAIN, NO PAIN ANYWHERE, NO PAIN IN MY BACK, STOMACH, RIBS, NOWHERE!!!! — OH YEEEAH!" 👍👍 (*Please, God, if only we could preserve in bottles those precious feelings and happy days and give them back to her later. I will remind her of such days.*)

She read me the medical report — clear abdomen, kidneys, pancreas, liver, gallbladder, no focal lesions, aortic, lymphoma. No fluid. Nodule on chest (lung) 1 cm, considerably smaller than four months ago, the Murphy test, called Murphy Sign*- no evidence of metastasis. Heart fecal normal. The prescriptions she is taking are:

(all*)	Metoprolol Tartrate	25 mg	¼
	Ondansetron	(nausea)	
	Acyclovir	400 mg	2X day
	Backarac	(bowel movements)	
	Trasodone	(sleep aid)	
	Omeprazole	stomach	
	Fluconazole		
	Gabapenpin	100 mg	2X day
	Potassasium	7 days	
	Magnesium	Medicare doesn't cover (We paid for the pills.)	
	Pain patches	Medicare doesn't cover (Her father had boxes of them and gave them to her.)	

9/20/10, Mon., Debra's call at 8:30 p.m.

Debra talked to Charron at RPCI; she asked if the CT scan and the medical reports that she had been given were sent to Dr. LaiLai. Charron told her that the doctor will be at Amherst all week but that he would get the information. When Debra was in ICU in isolation at NFMMH, one of the patients in another room was crying out "I want to die; I want to die." Her nurse came in to Debra's room in the middle of the night for blood or something and said: "That kind of upsets me so; here you are fighting for your life, and she wants to die."

I told Deb, "You've shown so much strength this year. You've been through so much, you've taken everything they have done to you and accepted it. You need to take a moment to thank God for this."

She said, "Yes, Mom, I have been talking to Him. I told Him, 'I'm not questioning why You are doing this to me, but I've been good for almost 17 years, I've straightened out my life, I have a son who is the light of my life, and I need to be here for him. I don't want what happened to his dad happen to him without a mother. I can't do that to him.' "

You need to keep doing that, Debra. Do you realize that the news you got was two days after Tia Connie (our 95- year old aunt in California) had been on a pilgrimage to the mission in New Mexico? I have the holy dirt and haven't even had a chance to rub it on you!" We were laughing, and because I had given her a small envelope of the "holy dirt", she said put in on! ⚓⚓

Personal: Debra called so excited, she couldn't believe it! Lisa and Doug have a mammoth garden (field), so Debra went on the side of house, she started pulling a few weeds out and underneath them, she found dozens of orange Japanese lanterns! "Mom, this was a gift of memory from my childhood because we had dozens of them around our house and inside our house! Do you remember? I do! I remember them!" So she and Lisa transplanted the lanterns in the front of the house in the circle garden which had a fountain, and then said "I hope they will keep." (*I used to dry the lanterns and use them in arrangements.*)

Personal: She and Donna went to the Halloween store and Deb found two wigs, they were baseball caps with real hair, one blond and one brown. Chris is taking her to the store on Tuesday to get them. "Mom, these will be OK for now." (*Oh, Debra, sweetheart.*)

9/28/10, Tues. —

This is Jeremy's birthday. We sent him a "Happy birthday, sweetheart" message. Hopefully, we'll see him this weekend.

10/6/10, Wed. —

Debra went to her pain management doctor in Amherst. Lisa was supposed to drive her, but at the last minute, she called her father. The pain doctor gave her injections in her back which has been hurting for a week, but she doesn't think it's anything from the chemo or the shingles.

She hasn't heard from Charron in Dr. LaiLai's office; all she gets are voice mail messages.

10/7/10, Thurs. —

Debra is awaiting a call from her new case worker; the one she liked probably left. I said, "Debra, if there's a new person, she's probably overwhelmed."

Personal: Donna thinks her own surgery is scheduled in November. Deb was in bed. I told her Jeremy's birthday card was still here. Debra told me Jeremy's dad and wife have been moving into a new house and have been very busy. She didn't even see Jeremy this weekend — his birthday.

Later, she called that she had talked to Charron; Dr. LaiLai hasn't even looked at her records or her CT scan. Charron informed Debra that she should prepare to get chemo next Thursday. (*Why? To compare the records to the one RPCI took in July.*) She's almost out of medication for the shingles and none of her prescriptions can be refilled. I told Debra that the doctor who ordered it should be the one who orders the refill.

10/14/10, Thurs. —

Upstate delivers Hydroc/ACET, Emend 125-80 mg, Docusate* 100 mg. Venlafaxine ER 75 mg, Omeprazole DR 20 mg, Trazodone 50 mg (*This is strange, why?*), Gabapentin 100 mg, Ondansetron 4 mg.

10/14, 15, 16/10 - Chemo Procedure: Cisplatin.

10/14/10, Thurs. — @ RPCI Amherst

Debra was to be examined and talk to doctor (not LaiLai), but he ended putting her on chemo for five hours! (*What happened?*) Debra now said that she didn't want to walk around knowing that she had a spot (however tiny) on her lung. She wanted to be told she was cancer-free. Next appointment is 11/4 at 8:00 a.m. and hopefully, it will be her last. She wants to be told that she was cancer-free.

Jerr and I ate lunch at the Grateful Deli. Debra did not want lunch or anything to eat. She said even the smell of food was nauseating her. Later she asked for a pain pill and took another anti-nausea pill. She called Chris to pick her up on his way home from work.

When we arrived back home, I went for a walk around our complex and picked the largest, most brilliant autumn leaves and wrapped a plant stem around them and gave Debra the mini-bouquet of leaves. She got a little smile on her face and just kept looking at the bouquet. "Mom, remember when you and Jeremy were jumping and rolling in the leaves?" *"Yes, sweetheart, I sure do."*

Personal: Today when Chris came home, he immediately fell asleep on the couch. Ginny comes over a couple times a day now I advised Deb to try putting positive thoughts in Ginny's head like how she used to paint (She's a wonderful portrait artist) and now she has the freedom to take it up again. That she (Debra) would look forward to seeing her work or to see her get involved with her church; to join a professional woman's group, or start developing friends in her area now that she can.

About Donna, Debra can use her food stamps to get her Ensure at Walgreen's because they are both going to be taking it. We made plans to go tomorrow morning.

10/15/10, Fri., 11:30 p.m. —

Debra was going to spend the day with us, possibly go to RPCI Buffalo to pick out a wig.

10/16/10, Sat. —

Debra went to stay with Ginny overnight; she said she already had her bag packed anyway. Ginny was very appreciative because she didn't want to stay alone, she said Deb was more understanding.

10/17/10, Sun. —

Such a joyful service at St. Gregory's. It is like my home, I get such solace there and such peace. It is an exceptional church. When I am not able to attend church or when we are in Florida, I am able to watch the services on the Internet.

10/18/10, Mon. —

Personal: Chris took the week off to take Ginny to handle all the personal financial changes. Debra thinks Tom has already been cremated. Later, Ginny will have a Mass said for him at church.

10/20/10, Wed. —

Debra feels stuffed up, like she had a cold, but that's one of the side affects of the chemo; she's not sniffling or sneezing. Taking ibuprofen 800 mg.

Personal: Last year, when Deb was first diagnosed, one of Chris' friends gave them a certificate for dinner at Salvatore's Italian Restaurant and a suite at their hotel, Garden Place. Chris found it had expired last Saturday, but Debra doesn't feel like going to have anything to eat especially at such a posh place. She called Salvatore's, and they stated they will honor the certificate for six months. In any event, they were all booked up this weekend. "Chris is really as wonderful person, Mom." "*I know, sweetheart.*"

10/22/10, Fri. —

Debra was so full of happiness; she called to tell us that on the Cash Cab program, she answered all the questions! Jerr said, "Wow! Let's do it for real; I'll take you to New York." Debra was laughing and said, "OK, that's a deal. Now how much money do you have for us to take all the cabs until we hit the Cash Cab?!" "Enough for you, girly, enough for you."

When Debra stayed with us, she and I would sit on the sofa and watch first Wheel of Fortune and then Jeopardy, our favorite. I could answer most of the question, but she could answer almost all of them. Jerr would just laugh at us and say, "Debra, you are a wonder. I'm amazed. Why don't you try out to be a contestant?" She answered, "Because I don't know the Greek gods and they ask a lot of those questions! Mom knows those better than me." (*We would have contests every time.*) 🛳 🛳 Jerr would just shake his head laughing.

Donna was with us because her GYN doctor is in our neighborhood. We had gone to Aldi's to buy what she needed. Deb had already done Donna's laundry, and she had dinner there. Then at 8:40 p.m., Deb called back and she said did not have a stomach pain because she was taking the generic Prilosec, so no heartburn. "Mom, it's wonderful, just a great feeling!"

Debra watched a TV special about Wings of Flight and stated that if she had the money, she would donate to them. The organization makes flights available to children and others when they need to get to a medical facility fast, and they do it at no charge. *Never heard of it, but do you mean Mercy Flight?* "Yes, yes, that's it; I would donate to them. Mom, if you got your pilot's license again, you could work with them, can't you? I remember when you were taking flying lessons and your boss was returning from an executive meeting with his staff in the corporate jet and they had to wait for you to land. They heard the announcement! You had never told him you were flying. Then later you took dad up when he didn't believe you could. It was so awesome.

"You've raised so much money for charity, that's what I'm going to do when I'm well. Let's work together at some of the places you did like The Salvation Army and dozens of others. Think of a favorite one that I can do and then I can make a difference, too." *We will, sweetheart.*

Regarding her ongoing car accident case five years ago: She has been referred her to the spine doctor, an orthopedic, who will help her with her Arbitration, however, that doctor still hasn't sent in the paperwork for her mileage of two years ago, he hasn't been paid almost $7,000 because he waited so long that it will now cost him $3,000 to go to court, he says!

10/27/10, Wed. —

Personal: Chris had a medical test today and he's sleeping; don't know if he will be coming tomorrow night. Talked about Donna's test, she may borrow Chris' car and she will drive the two of them.

11/2/10, Tues. —

A shopping trip to Wegmans where we bought loads of canned goods for Debra to take home — all her favorite vegetables, fruits, treats, and she stayed with us.

Upstate delivers Emend 125-80 mg, Venlafaxine ER 75 mg, Ondansetron 4 mg.

11/3, 4, 5/10 - Chemo Procedure: Cisplatin / Adriamycin.

11/4/10, Thurs. —

Today during her five-hour treatment, Debra wanted her usual egg salad sandwich. We deliver her lunch and return to the deli for ours.

11/18/10, Thurs. — @ MSMH

Debra called 911 at 7:00 a.m. and was taken by ambulance. She was admitted about 12:30 p.m., with a blood chemistry of 0.5 and very low potassium. They did a CT scan, and she was informed there was no sign of an infection so they couldn't give her antibiotics. (*She had been taking antibiotics for her abscessed tooth.*) The doctor also started her on blood transfusions again — A positive from an A positive donor. She didn't want to go to NFMMH because of how she was treated the last time she had to go; they didn't even take blood then.

Now she was so weak all day and all night, couldn't walk, she had a cough and wheezing; she couldn't even pull her pants down to use the bathroom. Jerr and I drove to Lewiston at 1:40 p.m. to see her and left about 8:00 p.m. It was dark black outside and pouring RAIN. It took us over one hour to get home.

Personal: Ginny comes over every night with "dinner" cooked so she can get praise from the boys and hear the boys say "Grandma, we don't have anything to eat." When Debra is able to make dinner, they don't eat it and snub their noses at it. She keeps trying to make their favorites. She said, "It really hurts especially because I'm trying so hard in spite of how I feel!"

Donna brought over her laundry for Debra to do, but Debra left it in the washing machine when she called 911.

I called Dr. LaiLai's Office; after passing through all the voice mails, I left a message about Debra's severe leg pains. Debra had been to the hospital night before and was given three pain shots and sent home. I can't believe that in that entire hospital, there isn't a doctor to prescribe Percocet or something that she needs. Charron called back very apologetic. Dr. LaiLai is out of town; she can't order anything, but Dr. Gadoy, his assistant, did call Upstate Pharmacy with the prescription of only 60 pills. Deb has to see her own pain management doctor. RPCI doctors stated that they can't understand why Deb is having these pains because it's not chemo related. I said, "Not true, Charron, it's a side affect of Cisplatin. Charron said, '**Deb's hasn't been given Cisplatin**". (*WHAT?! I looked on her schedules and she's had several Cisplatin infusions — on 9/16 and*

11/18/09! I told her we were so disappointed because we thought Deb was through with chemo and Laura at Amherst now told us she had eight more treatments.

Charron: "Eight? When you start a new therapy, you are back at square one. She must have misspoken because none of our therapies are eight; they are all six. Debra only has three more treatments left, and then Dr. LaiLai will order a CT scan and see where she is."

Deb called laughing and said, "Mom, you should be a negotiator for the United Nations!" Upstate Pharmacy delivered her prescription about 8:00 p.m.! Her next appointment with the pain management doctor is in January; she's not going to change it. I called Debra's health insurer and asked for a printout of her medical expenses (*never received them.*)

Donna was here because we were going to her GYN doctor for her appointment at 3:30 P.M. We again went to Aldi's for her groceries.

Then at 8:40 p.m., Deb called that she did not have stomach pain because she was taking the generic Prilosec again, so no heartburn. "Mom, it's wonderful!"

10/31/10, Halloween —

We didn't go the Pumpkinville in Clarence this year. For years we had taken Jeremy. There is a huge ruler there, and we always took Jeremy's picture of front of it, measuring how tall he had gotten from year to year. One year, he and his friend, our neighbor, had spent twenty minutes in line to get into the maze house. All of a sudden, Jeremy comes back to us and says, "Grandma, they won't let me in; they said I was too tall!" He was shocked. The maze house was one of his favorite attractions every year. Then, just this summer when we went to Canalfest, he wanted to go on the gigantic wheel where everybody stands up and the floor falls away as the wheel went faster and faster and tilted every which way. I was uncomfortable with this ride, but he was insistent because he said it looked so cool. Sure enough, after a few minutes, he returned to us very unhappy. He was told he wasn't big enough for the ride. I laughed and said, "Jeremy, that's life. Just like the story of the "Three Little Bears," remember? [And he looked at me as if to say, really, Grandma!] Some things are too big, some are too small and then there's the time when things are just right, and it's at that time that makes us so happy." We went on to ride the Tilt-A-Whirl though and the wheel ride was forgotten.

11/1/10, Mon. —

We sent a petition to the St. Jude Shrine for Debra.

11/2/10, Tues. —

We took a shopping trip to Wegmans where we bought loads of canned goods and other items for Debra to take home — all her favorite vegetables, fruits, treats.

11/4/10, Thurs. — Chemo Procedure: Adriamycin.

After Debra's treatment, she received a telephone message that the following morning, she was to have a telephone interview with a representative of Social Security. She now had to go home to get her files, and we drove her to Niagara Falls.

We had just returned home when Debra called and told us "OMG, Mom, I'm looking at the instructions, and I left my wallet in my hospital case at your house!" And in there, were all the ID cards she needed for next morning. So Jerr and I looked at each other, started laughing, got back in the car and returned to Niagara Falls with her wallet. Jerr, shaking his head with a smile on his face, "And this is what I raised these kids for?" It was 10:30 p.m. and we were nervous about driving there but we then spent another hour sitting in the car talking about a charity fundraiser Debra was going to attend and who the little boy was and what the family was experiencing without health insurance.

Debra tells Ginny to start painting again or join her church choir. "OMG, Mom, that reminds me of the weddings you used to sing and that love song you did. I always remembered it even when you would remind me if I had a spat with my boyfriend." "Yes, Debra, it was Corinthians in the Bible: *"Love is always patient and kind. It is never jealous. Love is never boastful or conceited. It is never rude or selfish. It does not take offense and is not resentful. Love takes no pleasure in other people's sins, but delights in the truth. It is always ready to excuse, to trust, to hope and to endure whatever comes."*

"OK, I've been told. Do you remember one of the operas you were in at the cathedral and I almost sat on the Bishop's lap?"

"Yes, you were with us downstairs in the dressing room and didn't go up the cathedral when the chimes rang. In your bright red spandex tights, your white silk blouse and spike heels, you got between us (the "hooded monks") processing into the darkened cathedral with dim candles -- and you saw an empty seat in the front row and went to sit down. That was the Bishop's reserved seat! And not only that, but when you turned into the row, the "monks" behind you started to turn in with you, and we had to pull their robe to stay back in our line along the side! OMG, a perfectly rehearsed staging almost ruined by a blonde chickie in red spandex! But the Bishop was so kind and pleasant to you when he found out I was in the opera and you were not someone set up to ACCOST him!"

"And, Mom, what about the opera when the tenor soloist raised his big toe every time he hit a high note and I could hardly stop from laughing."

"Yup, that was "The Bishop of Brindisi" and the tenor wore sandals with his robe. You had a 'legal' seat in the 2nd row and instead of focusing on the music, you were mesmerized with that big toe!" Which reminds me, Debra, I wish I had been able to sing at your wedding. When Phil came to me and knelt down and said he had asked you to marry him, I went out and bought a designer wedding dress for you. You said, you pick it out, and I'll wear it, I don't have the time or patience to shop!

"Mom, I'm so sorry that things didn't work out. Phil went off on his own when he got his huge settlement. I see that wedding gown in your closet, and I feel so sad at times. Then I think about Jeremy and at least I had that gift and nothing else matters." "And, Deb, I know that dress would not have been appropriate for the ceremony you guys had in mind."

11/5/10, Fri. —

Debra's appointment with Social Services; interview went well; her application will be approved; she has a new social director who's very nice!

Upstate delivers Omeprazole DR 20 mg, Trazodone 50 mg, Gabapentin 100 mg.

7:45 p.m. —

Debra is nauseated; the pills don't help; she been taking them every four hours. It's not bad enough to throw up; but just the awful feeling. She had a spoon of soup but then didn't want the rest. She tried rice, then pudding, then chicken; nothing appealed to her; she has no appetite. Debra said: "Mommy, you don't think RPCI is just doing this for money, do you?" (*Maybe — I haven't had a good feeling about them recently.*) She has been told that the lymph nodes have not shrunk. (I *thought they were taken out?*) She is going to call her health insurer for a copy of medical expenses paid on her behalf since she got sick in April 2009 and to date.

11/6/10, Sat. —

Took Donna to get cases of Walgreen's brand of Ensure. Which is the only brand that she could tolerate.

11/9/10, Tues. — "HAPPY BIRTHDAY, you big guy, Jerrrrrry! May you have many more." "He said, "Thanks, sweetheart, thank you for remembering." "Debra said, how could I forget, I've sooooooo many years to remember!" 🎂🎂

Upstate delivers Oxycodone 10 mg.

11/10/10, Wed. —

Debra has an abscessed tooth! I called our dentist and she was totally booked. I started calling dentists in Niagara Falls — finally after nine calls, found North Tonawanda Family Dentistry. The doctor gave her an appointment for the next day, Thursday, 10/11/10 at 8:00 a.m. "Mom, whew, what a relief." The doctor gave her a prescription for antibiotics. Her father will take her because Jerr has an appointment here for a fasting blood test at 8:30 a.m.

11/12/11, Fri., 6:45 a.m. —

Debra said she would take Donna for her 5:45 a.m. appointment for a colonoscopy* prior to her surgery. The endoscopy* will be performed at the same time. She called after the procedure and said it was no problem but she was diagnosed with diverticulitis, hiatal hernia* and ulcer! (*OMG, now what! What will the treatment be and with meds, we hope this will cure all her problems the poor girl has had over the years.*)

11/18/10, Thurs. —

We received a letter from Fr. Sticco of the St. Jude Shrine that "the petitions on behalf of Debra are being presented to St. Jude during our daily novenas." (*Please, God, accept the petitions from these holy men.*)

11/19/10, Fri., 11:30 a.m. @ MSMH in Lewiston —

Debra was admitted last night. She was awake all night with the IV machine beeping; the nurse kept coming in numerous times to reset it; every time the beep went off, she would start crying, it was like water torture. She said, "I'd rather be home, at least it's quiet for the most part." Finally the morning nurse reset the machine so it wouldn't go off and she fell asleep at 9:00 a.m. When we saw her, her eyes were all swollen from crying and no sleep. No doctors have been in to see her yet this morning and they haven't said anything about going home. She had another bag of blood transfusion for a total of two so far, her potassium was low, and she was given a bag of platelets.

11/20/10, Sat., 10:00 a.m. —

Doctors have not been in today as yet; she only received the bag of platelets yesterday, no more blood transfusions.

Upstate delivers Acetaminophen.

Deb's tooth pain has come back; her cheek is starting to puff out; asked me to call her dentist, Dr. Pabney. The office hours are open week days and today is Saturday but the recording said: "In emergencies, call Dr. Pabney's cell phone. So I did. Dr. Pabney was so surprised to receive a call as she was at a dental clinic at an Army camp in upstate New York. She said she didn't know how the call came through because they are very strict about cell phones, were not to receive calls and the reception was poor! Dr. Pabney needed the pharmacy phone number and the name of the prescription. I told her Debra couldn't fight the infection because she was in the hospital. Debra said she'll get the information from Chris and call me, and then I'll call the doctor back. At 11:00. Debra called to tell me she asked Chris to get the information and he said he was busy with his mother. Deb started crying that he couldn't even do this one simple thing for her. We finally got the information and the dentist called the prescription in for an antibiotic, Clindamycin, 150 mg, 2 every 6 hrs. Dr. Pabney's associate was Dr. Sachteva.

3:00 p.m. —

Debra called to tell us not to come to the hospital; the doctor was discharging her and she was going home; she'll call me when she gets home.

11/21/10, Sat. — Donna's Pre-Op prior to surgery at MFSH —

We arose at 7:00 a.m. Donna had an appointment at 8:30 a.m. for her pre-op tests prior to her hysterectomy surgery. Jerr had to be at the cardiologist at 9:40 a.m. Donna never arrived until 9:30 after experiencing one personal emergency after another; she will go directly to the hospital and we will meet her there. After Jerr's appointment, we sat in the waiting room until she was finished at 11:30 a.m. Then we went to the Cracker Barrel for brunch and came home.

11/24/10, Wed. —

MY BIRTHDAY CARD

Mom, you've given me so much. I look around
and see so many unhappy people who don't seem
to believe in themselves or feel worthy of what
they want…or have. And I can't help but wonder
if they'd had a mom, like you, how different
their lives might be, how much more confidence
they might have, how many more of their hopes
could have become realities. Your love, time, and
support were priceless gifts. Every day these gifts
are with me in the joys I feel, the challenges I face,
and the dreams I follow. And every day I think of
you with appreciation and so much love. Thank
you for my life. I love you. Debra & Jeremy.

11/25/10, Thurs. — **THANKSGIVING** —

Donna was not feeling well and couldn't eat anything; she was really sick. Our families were going to Samuel's Grand Manor for Thanksgiving dinner. It would be a waste for her to go. The seven us of went together, Sammy and Faye, Mark and Sally, Jerr and Debra and me.

Personal: Debra's going to come over Wednesday night and stay for Thanksgiving dinner. Chris will pick her up on Friday. He felt he had to be with his mother this holiday. Then next week, she'll do it again for her chemo.

11/26/10, Fri. — Donna's birthday —

I called Donna at 7:15 a.m. to wish her a happy birthday, "old lady"! Over the years, I always wanted to be the first to say "Happy Birthday" to the girls.

(The Spaniards have a beautiful traditional song to wish someone "Happy Birthday" early in the morning — it's called "Mananitas." And is sung quietly with a guitar.)

Upstate delivers Lorazepm 1 mg.

11/27/10, Sat. —

Chris stopped on Grand Island at the guitar store, and he and Debra had a good talk about the boys and what Chris wants them to do around the house to share chores. Chris is home this week and he said things are going to change.

I called for Debra's prescription, she only has two refills. The appointment with the pain management doctor is not until January. The other girl told Debra that they filled her prescription as a one-time courtesy basis only and can't do it again. They will give it to me if I can pick it up.

I called Dr. LaiLai's office, (Charron); there was a mix up in Debra's prescription.

Debra went to the dentist and to Walgreen's.

Debra told me that when she was looking for Christmas decorations, she found her pay stubs from Country Glen. She laughed because she started out at minimum wage and had received small raises. With this amount, she paid her rent of $350 and all her utilities, drove to Buffalo to pick up Jeremy, then get his special groceries, and make sure he has special gifts. But you know, Mommy, I am so proud of myself for doing this on my own, taking care of Jeremy (with your help, of course) and doing whatever it takes to have Jeremy. He's my life. I'll do anything. We have fun."

11/29/10, Mon., 6:45 a.m., Donna's surgery at MFSH

Donna stayed with us overnight. We greeted the day at 6:00 a.m.; surgery was scheduled for 9:00 a.m. She was taken to pre-op at 9:20 a.m. I was allowed to accompany her. Then the doctors were very concerned that her potassium was very high. They asked if she had eaten a lot of bananas (*no*). After a delay, a second test indicated the levels were now normal and preparation was started for her surgery. Her doctor told us that he will see us in 1-½ hours. We were given her patient number which would be displayed on an electronic board in the waiting room. Four and a half hours later, the board kept showing "IN OR", "IN OR", the volunteer informed us, "Don't leave the area, the doctor will want to see you." *Oh, my God, I prayed, please let everything be OK.*

Finally 5-½ hours later, the doctor came out and said, "Would you come with me please?" I asked, "Oh, we can finally see her?" He said, "No, I'd like to talk to you privately in this room."

(*I was gripping Jerr's hand. Oh, God, please God, she has been so sick; do not let the biopsy reveal another cancer and let this be the solution to her problems. I was terrified. I was feeling ice cold. We followed the doctor.*)

In the consultation room, the doctor told us, "I've been doing this for numerous years, and this was one of the most difficult surgeries I have ever done. We started out with lapriscope, went in through the belly button and on the right side, and everything went normal, a piece of cake. Then I inserted the probe on the left side and couldn't get it in, I tried and tried and finally we said abort, prepare for surgery, and once I could see what was happening, I saw all her bowels were stuck together, they were stuck to the uterus, to the ovaries, and even to the side wall of her belly. I literally had to peel them apart. I got everything out; she has nothing left. The good news is there was no sign of cancer, the biopsies were normal. (*Thank you, Jesus, thank you.*) She's in recovery, will probably take quite a while because we had to keep pumping her with anesthetic for the duration of the surgery. She's been assigned a room, and as soon as we take her upstairs; we'll take you up." We returned to the waiting room and I was sobbing.

After another two hours, we were taken to Donna's room. We found her in such pain and asking for pain meds! She felt like the left side was ripping, right side was OK. She was drinking liquids. (Was *this going to be a repeat of a nightmare?!*) The nurse said she would probably sleep now, that we didn't need to wait. I informed her that we wanted to wait! After Donna had fallen asleep, we still remained for two hours and then came home. (*I cried my eyes out for my little peanut, my sweetie. But I prayed that all her problems would be resolved at last!*)

11/30/10

Upstate delivers Emend 125-80 mg.

12/1/10

Upstate delivers Omeprazole DR 20 mg, Ondansetron 4 mg

12/2/10, Thurs. —

We could not visit Donna but I called several times throughout the day, and planned to stop and see her that evening. She had taken her sketch book to the hospital. We were with Debra at chemo center for five hours.

12/2/10, Thurs. — Chemo Procedure: Cisplatin.

12/3/10, Fri. — Donna's discharge from hospital —

Donna woke us up at 7:40 a.m., said doctor was there and was going to discharge her; he was calling for someone to remove her staples! (*Yikes, ouch.*) She will call when she's ready as it usually it takes about five hours, but at 8:30, she was ready!

I awoke Debra as she was returning home, and we left to pick up Donna at the hospital. I wanted her to stay with us but she said she needed to get back to her dogs. We stopped at the pharmacy to get her prescriptions en route to Niagara Falls. When we got her home, it was an experience getting her up the stairs and keeping the dogs from greeting her! Initially, Donna told us she would stay with her father, getting up only to let the dogs out, and when she felt she wanted to go home, that Debra would help her with the stairs. I planned to buy groceries and return the next day.

12/5/10, Sun. —

This is the beginning of the Advent season in the Catholic church. It is so exciting that in spite of the dire messages in the readings of the gospel, the underlying message is hope. My prayer at church today is that Debra be given hope, in her life, in her treatments, and for her future. And for Donna's recovery and hope that this surgery will fix what has been making her sick every day. *Oh, healing Jesus, I place my daughters in Your hands.*

12/15/10, Wed. —

Personal: Called Debra because Donna was back at her apartment! I thought she was with her father? Debra said everything changed. "Let us know what she needs, Debra, we'll take care of it."

12/20/10, Mon. —

"Mom, you cannot get here today; there's three feet of snow, I cannot drive Chris' new car in this snow and there was a travel advisory for all unnecessary travel. Donna has been to Doug's, and Jim came over, but I took her shopping for food, paid for her prescriptions and bought her food for her two dogs."

On Christmas Day, Debra has to pick Jeremy up because he is at Phil's; but don't know what will happen.

Personal: Chris is making lasagna for Christmas Day and his brother and sister-in-law are coming over. Debra doesn't even know how she's going to be feeling after her chemo on the 23rd. The driving is so bad that Chris doesn't get home from Buffalo until 5:30 instead of 3:30.

Debra is so excited. She called to tell me that on 12/27, HGTV are going to feature the prize-winning Christmas houses in the Village of Youngstown and two Canadian houses. There will also be a re-run in a few days. Also, Debra said that on 12/23, which should be her last chemo, instead of us ordering the fruit baskets for the nurses at RPCI, she can buy a fruit basket at Wegmans and take it with her! She only hopes she can make it with the snow.

Upstate delivers Hydrocodone*, Gabapentin* 100 mg, Avelox* 400 mg, Fluconazole* 200 mg, Acyclovir 500 mg.

12/18/10, Sat. —

We called Debra and she didn't answer her phone or call back; she must have gone home.

12/23/10

Upstate delivers Emend 125-80 mg.

Chemo Procedure: CPK Chemo

12/24/10, Fri., 6:30 p.m. —

Debra received a message from RPCI about January 13 - but no reason what that is about and no explanation as to reason for the appointment? We were led to believe that this Thursday was to be her last chemo treatment. She had her treatment and when she was finished, the nurses didn't applaud her like they have other patients who completed their treatments. She should be finished. She's going to call on Monday and find out what is going on.

Personal: "Mommy, whew; I just got home; so tired; went to the Boulevard Mall shopping; was up last night until 1:00 a.m. decorating the tree, trying to do my magic with this poor tree; it looks all right but no comparison with the trees you used to do. Tonight, Chris and I will watch the Christmas Story, we do this every year; we love it; it's about the little boy, Ralphie, who got a pellet gun — since he loved the hero in the Westerns from the 50's — shoots it and it breaks his glasses; he lied and said an icicle did it.

"Tomorrow we're going to dad's; Donna cooked a mini-lasagna and cheesecake; I didn't want to be here at Chris' house with his brother and sister-in-law and the kids coming over, and Ginny with all her crying that it's the first Christmas without Tom. The streets are clear but it's very cold. I pick up Jeremy tonight; it will be so exciting to have Christmas with him."

She didn't ask me but I told her I was getting ready to go to Midnight Mass; that's the "Reason for the Season". I asked her to take a moment to say "thank you", because she has a lot to be thankful this year. She said, "Yes, I do, Mom, truly. There are many, many times when I can't sleep at the hospital or here at home and that's all I think about — our religion and what brought me to this time. Merry Christmas, Mom. And I love you two, too," *"Debra, we love you, too, God bless you, sweetheart."*

12/17/10, Fri. @ NFMMH —

In the evening, Debra had another angel of a nurse, Dawn. When Debra mentioned that her mouth was so dry she couldn't even talk, the nurse brought her sponge tubes that looked like popsicles on a tiny stick, and they smelled like spearmint. Dawn looked like Patty Duke and wore a black leather headband-Debra loved her! Dawn did some online research on the Internet for us and printed about six pages regarding the side effects from chemo. I can't help but wonder: "Why did RPCI not give Debra this information -- or any other information about the soothing products, about those oral swabs, or skin care products like Dawn Mist?" Debra said, "Even after washing my face, I can rub my fingers across my forehead and skin would roll off!" She always said the three "Bs" really worked: Be nice to everybody because you'll never know if they'll be your Boyfriend, your Boss or your Best friend! She remembered, "There was a dummy-looking, bumbling guy at work; everybody made fun of him except me, Mom. I would go out of my way to ask him questions or just say a word to him. Then one day he was promoted as their Production Line Supervisor and guess who he was nice to? Me, Mom, not the girls who had made fun of him!"

Deb called back and said, "Let's watch 'Charlie Brown's Christmas program together; I love it, Mom. Do you remember when the three of us would watch it together?" So I turned it on and after the program, we laughed and talked about it. How funny it still was and how we could appreciate the message as adults.

Later in the evening, "Mom, watch HGTV on Thursday at 8:00 p.m.; they are going to re-run the Christmas house decoration program with houses from Youngstown and Niagara Falls.

12/24/10 - Christmas Eve —

Went to Midnight Mass, prayed for my husband, daughters, grandson, all our families and friends. If only the quiet magic of Christmas could touch and change all of our hearts and souls.

12/25/10 - Christmas Day

I read Debra a card we received from Father Dominic at Sacred Heart Monastery — a poem by Wilda English:

> God grant you the light in Christmas, which is faith;
>
> the warmth of Christmas, which is love;

the radiance of Christmas, which is purity;

the righteousness of Christmas, which is justice;

the belief in Christmas, which is truth;

the all of Christmas, which is Christ.

"Merry Christmas, my Debra; we love you." "Merry Christmas, Mummy; love you two, too."

12/26/10, Sun. —

Debra called from NFMMH, she felt very weak and sick, couldn't raise her arm up. She told Chris, "I feel like I did when I had to call 911." It was about 4-5:00 p.m. He asked if she wanted to go to the hospital. Debra told him, "Not yet, let's wait a while."

Then about 6-7 p.m., she said, "Chris, I'd better go, I'm feeling worse." When the blood tests were run, her white blood cells registered as "1" and they should have been 7-8! The E/R doctor told her, "We almost lost you." She was found to have a small infection in her tooth, and was started on blood transfusions and antibiotics. She called her dentist who said the antibiotics she is given in the hospital are stronger than what she could prescribe. Debra was so excited because she had, Monique, an older woman with short, gray hair, an angel of a nurse, who was in her room with her meds every two hours; she didn't even have to call for her pain shots. Her doctor, a Indian oncologist; is very nice, very tall.

Personal: Her father is very sick; he was supposed to heat the oven and cook ham for Christmas. When Debra and Donna got to his house, he was asleep in bed, the ham was still frozen, and the kitchen was a mess. Donna had baked a mini-lasagna and a small cheesecake; they just stored it at his house and left. Donna went to Doug's and Debra went back to Chris'. She had Jeremy with her. Ginny gave her a pair of soft lounging pants. It was quiet Christmas.

2011

THE CONTINUING TREATMENTS

1/4/11 - Chemo Procedure scheduled: Cisplatin. No chemo today or tomorrow — Debra is to call RPCI.

1/6/11, Thurs. —

Debra is going to have a dental cleaning on 1/11; an extraction on the 17th and dental implants on the 31st.

1/7/11, Fri. — @ E/R NFMMH —

Chest pain, shortness of breath, nausea, vomiting, diarrhea or temperature over 100.4°. Finally discharged with instructions to continue Prilosec, Lortab, CBC in 3 days, and call primary doctor.

1/9/11, Sun. —

Good luck on Thursday. "Mom, here's a list of my prescriptions, do you think you can type a card for me to take to doctors with me? I know what they are, but you made up a really nice form for Jerr's meds. The doctors love you!"

Debra's Prescriptions:

Ondansetron	4 mg	Nausea from chemo

Gabapentin	100 mg	Nerve pain / shingles
Trazodone	50 mg	Antidepressant
Omeprazole	20 mg	Stomach / esophagus / heartburn
Acyclovir	400 mg	Anti-fungal — discontinue when finished
Venlafaxine	75 mg	
(Effexor/Zoloft)	100 mg	Constipation / diarrhea
Ondansetron	4 mg	Nausea — discontinue
Fluconazole	200 mg	
Metoprolol	25 mg	Discontinued

Personal — There was a blizzard, Debra was stranded at her father's and now there's been another blizzard going on. Debra has a lot going on this coming week. She's having her teeth cleaned on Monday, tooth extracted on the 25th, whew!

Personal: Debra had a discussion with Chris about the fact that she has to sleep at her friend, Lisa's house. It's closer for Debra and Lisa to get to the chemo center by 9:00 a.m., whereas Chris has to be at work by 5:00 a.m. and can't continue to take days off. Chris' house is in the opposite direction from the chemo center, and it would take Lisa 30-40 minutes to pick her up and then come all the way back.

1/10/11

Upstate delivers Emend 125-80 mg, Venlafaxine ER 75 mg, Omeprazole DR 20 mg.

1/13/11, Thurs. —

Chemo treatment — MY LAST ONE, MUMMY?? 🛁🛁

1/14/11, Fri. and 1/15/11, Sat. —

Debra called, finally talked to her later; she missed her chemo treatment; she couldn't sleep all night and was awake until 5:00 a.m. When the alarm rang at 7:00, she just couldn't get up, she just couldn't. She called RPCI and they couldn't reschedule her for this coming Thursday, so they split her appointments up, Wednesday (downtown) to see doctor and Friday at Amherst. She said she could probably drive herself to Buffalo if she could get on the highways.

(*Talked to Charron who gave Debra erroneous information again;* said she hadn't gotten the message Debra had left on the voice mail at 7:30 a.m.)

1/24/11, Mon. —

Debra made an appointment with the dentist who called Dr. LaiLai about her treatment. Had to reschedule it in about 3 weeks because Dr. LaiLai hasn't called/faxed dentist to inform her about how to treat Debra. She has to get her blood tested the day before and have them fax the results to the dentist.

More snow; it's 5° outside; difficult to get to treatments. Occasionally she feels pain, weak, stiff — went to hospital; she knew she had to go because of low blood count; she felt so weak she couldn't move.

"Mom, 'Housewives of Miami' are filming from Miami and South Beach; we see familiar landmarks!"

Personal: Mom, Donna needed a supply of bottled water; we went to the grocery store; her apartment is now neat and clean, all the papers gone. The bedroom is going to be her studio. We're going though all her clothes and discarding articles to donate. The sofa cover is all tucked in. I am taking her lunch."

Personal: (very upset) "Guess what, Mom? Ginny called Chris to meet her after work and the two of them bought furniture for living room — a huge brown sofa, two recliners, a love seat — all brown material and both chairs go into recliners with huge high backs plus a new table glass for the TV. Then for the upstairs bedroom new lamps. Back to the living room, the gold shade lamps look like toilet paper and make the living room real dark. There's barely any room to walk between all the huge furniture in this tiny room. The rugs are still a dirty pink and that's what we needed more than furniture! Chris is so happy because he's never had new furniture. He falls asleep on one side; Ginny falls asleep on the other side." Debra stays in her room. Debra was really hurt, so the furniture she and Chris were supposed to shop for is out. She had even made a schematic and measured the room. "Mom, the two of them didn't even ask my opinion. This furniture is overwhelming. So what am I doing here — for nine years?!" ⚲ L

1/31/11, Mon., 11:20 a.m. —

Tooth extraction at North Tonawanda Family Dentistry. Dr. Sachdeva was wonderful to her. She said that it was so easy and didn't even feel the pinch of Novocain.

2/1/11, Tues. —

An RPCI Community Volunteer Specialist acknowledged a donation in Debra's name. We were informed that the squares will be joined to make blankets for the patients. (While we were going through this cancer experience, one of our best Florida friends, Linda, began knitting classes for the "Sorority Sisters" of the Library in our Florida condo. They all made squares in a lovely assortment of colors and they were sent to RPCI. The Library Group is a group of women and men who began meeting at 9:30 p.m. in the library on the 1st Floor. This allowed us to fulfill all obligations, dinner, shopping, theater, etc. and were finished between 9:30 and 11:00 p.m.. Over the years, we have had anywhere from eight and more people stop in. We have shared lots of laughter, silliness, tears, problems, joys, births and deaths, medical challenges and feeling gratitude for good medical reports. We've shared childhood memories, school/college experiences, work, politics, religions — every facet of our lives. We've mourned the death of dear friends and rejoiced at the birth of grandchildren.)

2/5/11, Sat. —

Debra got a letter from RPCI that she had missed her treatment and appointment with Dr. LaiLai. WHEN WAS IT??? Never got a schedule; never got a follow-up phone call. It was to have been on 2/2 and 2/10. Now, they are going to "fit her in" at 6:00 p.m. at RPCI (Buffalo? She has to find a ride there — no one wants to go into Buffalo at night and in that area and parking lot! Radiology didn't tell her what to do for the CT scan; but she knew she was to have nothing to eat — but from the night before, or the morning, or when? Debra said she felt RPCI was like a factory — get 'em in; get 'em out. No personal touch; no comforting words, no information — at least not to her — but then she doesn't have the money that others do who are catered to. She changed her appointment.

2/10/11, Thurs. —

Debra saw Dr. LaiLai who said the module in her lung was minimized to the size of a pen dot (i) but he wants her to go for three more treatments beginning next week. Then in between those weeks, he will do another CT scan. She asked about the scheduled dental work? He answered, "No, it's on hold for now." When Debra has her blood test next week, she'll ask the office to fax the results to her dentist and make an appointment for Friday for the cleaning and go from there. She feels good about the fact that all the stomach cancer is gone and that it didn't spread anywhere else. It could have gone anywhere. But she and the doctor want to know that everything is gone. She was so happy about that, and we laughed that she was seeing an end to all this. "Yeeeaaaah," she laughed. 🔨🔨

Upstate delivers Emend 125-80 mg, Dexamethasone 4 mg.

2/18/11, Fri. — Chemo Procedure: Cisplatin.

2/19/11, Sat. —

Debra called; she had her chemo treatment yesterday; nurses were so happy to learn that her stomach cancer was GONE and that there was only one small dot in her lung, requiring only three more treatments — so she had her treatment today, on March 10 and possibly March 31st. Then three weeks after, will have another CT scan and God willing, she should be done!

She said she thinks her happy, positive attitude came from the last time she saw Dr. LaiLai, and he came in the room smiling and shaking her hand and said how happy he was that her stomach cancer was gone. "My gosh, Mom, he actually spent a moment with me." She keeps remembering that statement. After two years, finally a positive comment. She dreams of hearing that statement. She thanks God for that statement! She has practically eliminated all her pills, only takes a pain pill occasionally, not every four hours as directed — a Prilosec for her stomach. Now she's down to one or two pain pills and the Prilosec. She asks, "Is RPCI just in it for the money; they could make money on her Medicaid." RPCI Clinic combined the diuretic with the chemo and she was finished in only three hours — they gave her azithromycin*. She had no side effects from this the last time and today she felt only slightly tired, but good so far.

At Lisa's yesterday, she fell asleep until Lisa came and woke her up for dinner. Today, she said, "I could lie down but I'm not going to. Doctors did a heart test downstairs like they did four months ago and that test and my blood chemistry was good." She stayed at Lisa's an extra day because her prescriptions were due and she picked them up at the corner pharmacy instead of coming home and then going out there again.

Personal: *I informed Debra that because of their late notice, I was having a problem making their plane reservations for Florida. The cost this year* was extremely high because it was spring break and Easter falling so close together. Debra said, "Mom, don't worry about it; we can go next year." We offered a trip to New York City this summer instead, and she said, "Although Jeremy will be disappointed about the Florida trip, he would probably be more excited about NYC instead. Jeremy's playing football with the Warriors now; they have games every Sunday; he's a defensive linebacker (which protects the quarterback) *(So — I didn't know!)* Some of the games will be on TV and if their team wins, they will be playing at the Buffalo Bills' Rich Stadium. She was so excited and hoped he could have that experience! ⚓ ⚓

2/24/11 —

Upstate delivers Omeprazole DR 20 mg

2/28/11, Mon. @ E/R NFMMH —

Debra called that she has a severe sore throat; has been there since Saturday night; her face is swollen, her eyes are swollen, she's dehydrated, needs fluids; very low magnesium. In the midst of all this in the E/R, a girl came in asking her for $14 cash for the TV and was so rude to her because she was talking to me on the phone and then reached up and flipped the TV off. Debra was crying; she told the girl she had never had to pay for the TV. Later, a little woman about 80 years of age told Debra she overheard the girl and said she was going to report it. *(Angels.)*

3/3/11, Thurs. @ NFMMH —

She was finally started on blood transfusions at 11:00 p.m., her nurse said she didn't know why they waited so long to give it; waited all day for doctor to come in. During the night, her temperature went up to 104°, and it was finally brought down to 99°. Hospital does not want to send her home, only to have a problem develop, and she has to come back and have IVs inserted all over again. Doctors there are reluctant to do anything; let someone else (*RPCI?*) give the orders and then they carry them out. A nice Jewish doctor with gorgeous teeth (bling 🦷) and smile came in. He doesn't know why she isn't responding to the blood transfusions; it is not raising the blood count; it is not holding steady; it keeps going down. Doctor has talked to Dr. LaiLai who gave him a few options to try. S/B 17,000 and it's only 12,000.

3/4/11, Fri., 3:31 p.m. @ NFMMH —

She is getting another bag of blood; oncologist said he's not going to send her home until she's better. Nurse said she could go into the waiting room to watch TV; she came and brought her a blanket and pillow; then later stated, "You have 20 minutes before your next pain shot; do you need one, Debbie?" "God, yes, just sitting in that horrible, uncomfortable bed or this chair, my back is killing me. Here you are trying to save my life and Channel 21 in my room is going to kill me!" It's a local channel and plays one thing over and over and over again. (*Angels.*)

Debra's speech is slurred; she has a cut on her tongue from her abscessed tooth; she is being given antibiotics. Dr. Amend from RPCI ordered Cipro for a bladder infection. "Mommy, how can I possibly have a bladder infection since I'm so careful at home and at your house with my personal wipes?" I told her possibly it was the medicines coming out. (*What do I know? Why isn't she being given information?*) Web MD has become my daily Internet search. That site is where we've gotten most of our information.

Last week, Thursday, Debra had to be at RPCI at 8:00 a.m., then at 8:30, they did the heart test, couldn't find a vein, tried twice. She was crying. Then she sat upstairs until 12:30 p.m. to be examined by the doctor; and they finally left about 1:00 p.m.! Dr. LaiLai was very friendly, smiling, said he had taken a few days off. As a consequence, all his appointments were backed up. Deb said "You can't do that, Dr. LaiLai." He just laughed. "My, God, Mom, maybe all he needed was a vacation, but how do these doctors take vacations when treatments are so scheduled?"

I told Debra "I blame myself a thousand times for not making sure you were going for your yearly checkups. We talk about everything, Debra, why not this?" She responded, "Mom, I'm an adult; I felt good, was never sick in my life so thought there wasn't any need to go for my yearly tests, until I started bleeding. I told Donna that maybe I'm just going into early menopause. I know my smoking all those years ago didn't help me either. I regret what I did. I know it's my fault, Mommy. I just thought I was invincible. Why do young women think they are invincible?"

"Debra, I'm going to tell you something I remember from one of the seminars I conducted: Don't let your regrets have that much power. Don't let them have that much space. Take what "should have been" out of the picture and put HOPE in its place. Let's just hope for the best and hope that doctors know what they are doing and hope that the treatments will enable you to recover — and that's my prayer, too, sweetheart."

I love you, Mummy, you always give me such peace. *"I love you, too, Debra. My words are all I have in this situation. I feel so helpless; I can't control what is happening to you, and I can't control what's being done to you, You're my little princess, and I pray that God in His mercy will heal you."*

Personal: Jeremy practiced at the Buffalo Bills facility (indoors); he was excited.

Personal: She was so excited! Chris purchased a couple of magazines to read while she has her chemo. A Woman's Day article was about the author selling crafts online. There is no charge for setup or listing online — jewelry wonder.com — and sellers set their own prices. Another one was selling artwork.com; $10 Pro Account-pics (Donna knows how to access the Website) set up online store 20 per listing item, pay 3.5% commission of sale. "Mom, can you look it up for me, that's what I want to do when I'm finished here. I can just see it and now that's all I can think about." (*Angels!*)

Her doctor is Dr. Mohamad Ismail (bling).

3/10, 11, 12/11 - Chemo Procedure: Cisplatin.

3/15/11, Tues. —

Debra is sorry she didn't return my calls; her phone charger was at Chris' house and her battery ran out. She stayed at Lisa's and Doug's over the weekend to watch the dogs-two pit bulls, real nice — (*really?*) while they attended a snowmobiling event in Lake Placid. Lisa wanted to pay her for staying there. I told Debra, "Tell Lisa, OK, you can pay me for dog sitting, but then I will pay you for driving me to Amherst and to Buffalo for all my chemo treatments!" We laughed. ☝☝

Upstate delivers Emend 125-80 mg.

3/23/11

Upstate delivers Omeprazole DR 20 mg

3/24, 24, 25/11 - Chemo Procedure: Cytoxan*. (*This is a new one, why the change?*)

4/7/11, Thurs., 4:00 a.m. @ E/R MSMH —

Debra's in terrible stomach pain like an ulcer, a stabbing pain; her throat is raw and felt closed up like something was stuck there; couldn't swallow not even water. The doctor said she was full of white spots in the throat, into her esophagus; her immune system was down. E/R doctors called in a gastroenterologist who will check that there is no blockage in her esophagus; she was very thirsty but couldn't even swallow water or ice chips; she was started on antibiotics (*Could this be from the new chemo? Could this be from her infected molars again? She's at a standstill until she finishes chemo.*) She was started on PPI* (like for an ulcer?); but a few hours later, she was better, not in pain. Later, she ate a pulled pork sandwich and when she finally got to her room, they brought her a turkey sandwich, chicken noodle soup, broccoli and carrot cake and she ate everything; she was so hungry!

4/8/11, Fri. @ MSMH —

Doctor just came in and informed her that the gastro doctor will be in probably on Saturday. He will make arrangements to conduct the test as an outpatient later. "Mom, do you want to hear a good story? One of my favorite nurses, (she is like the girl from the Little House on the Prairie), saw me on the admission list; came in at 4:00 a.m. and got I a room at 3:30 p.m., Linda said, "sh sh, just between us, I overrode another patient so that you could get this room. The hospital is testing a new Sleep Number bed and you are the only one to have it!" "Mom, it is soooooo comfortable! My back doesn't hurt and you know how they always have to give me pain meds for the back pain? Well, I don't need them yet. See, one good turn does another one. I have angels around me. When I get my own apartment back, can we go shopping for a Sleep Number bed?" (*"Yes, of course, sweetheart."*)

Doctors are not adding to her pain meds; did an abdominal scan; something is pushing on gallbladder or her stomach; she won't eat but had a bowel movement yesterday, they tried to give her morphine, OxyContin. "Just wish it would stop hurting, Mommy." (*So do I. Please, God, what can I do? What is it that You want me to do for my daughter? I listen with my heart for Your message. I try to search my mind for a solution or course of action we can take.*)

4/9/11, Sat., 4:00 p.m. @ MSMH —

Debra not doing very well today; she has a fever, her chest hurts, given dose of antibiotics again last night in a glass bottle. The nurse said, "It's the first time I've given this in a glass bottle; don't know what kind of infection you have, Debra." Doctor will keep tabs on her fever; people say Deb is their "favorite patient". She barely laughed. Last night, her snack was peanut butter and jelly, fruit cup and milk. She is due to go to RPCI on Tuesday for blood work; she can drive herself and then if the numbers are OK, she goes for another chemo treatment on Thursday (*Please, God, her last one?*). MSMH did not notify Dr. LaiLai because her numbers are really good so it is not cancer-related. (*Well, then, what? What?*) I told them that he was on vacation anyway. Gastro doctor finally did a CT scan and found Deb has had **SHINGLES** for three weeks; she was at the tail end of it! (*OMG — again?*) A cardiologist wanted to admit her for her heart; pain med not touching it; no chemo; two days; infection in throat and esophagus — she was given Lyrica* 75 mg and antibiotics. Tests performed were a sonogram* and a MUGA* scan test on her heart.

Personal: "It's warm outside about 60, and it's supposed to get to 80 but then drop back to 40!" (*It doesn't matter, sweetheart, we are coming back from Florida.*) WHY???

Personal: "All the snow is gone with all the rain falling. We are getting a strange mini-blizzard, but then the snow is gone. TV weatherman said it was a good weekend to pick strawberries. Remember when we used to do that and when I've taken Jeremy? Must be why he has a strawberry birthmark on his neck! All those strawberries!" 😊😊

4/9/11, Sat., 5:00 p.m. @ MSMH —

The gastro doctor came in and said "Boy, you're in high demand around here, Debra!" He's going to talk to his supervisor and see if the test can be done on Monday instead of sending her home and then scheduling her for the test later. (*Angels, Mom.*) They don't know if it's a viral infection or some other kind. She may not be able to go to RPCI on Tuesday (the hospital called Charron.) "Mom, how can some doctors and nurses just make you feel so good especially when you're in pain and other people can stab you with their words and actions?" (*It happens in real life, too, sweetheart, even when a person is not sick. But you know, they probably have more problems than you do but you're lucky, you are getting help.)*

4/9/11, Sat., 9:15 p.m. @ MSMH —

The nurse told her the test is scheduled tomorrow (Sunday) at 3:00 p.m.! No food or drink after midnight, just sips of crushed ice; she will be given a sedative, then completely sedated in the Cath Lab, the doctor will put a scope down her throat and see what is there.

4/10/11, Sun., 2:00 p.m. @ MSMH —

I called her room, no answer. *(Please, God, let everything be alright.)*

4/10/11, Sun., 6:00 p.m. @ MSMH —

The scope test is done, laparoscopy ultrasound and camera; she was taken down before 2:00 p.m.; the doctor didn't come in until 3:30. She didn't feel a thing; he took biopsies, said everything looks good; he will let her know the results. The antibiotics they gave her may have started breaking the infection down. Afterward she was given broth, ice cream, juices, and a raspberry Popsicle — yummy! Then when she went to her room, she had a dinner of meat loaf, mashed potatoes, veggies, her favorite, and she is going to ask the dietician for more! "Mom, I always have angels around me. You're so right!"

4/11/11, Mon., 5:00 p.m. @ MSMH —

Debra is getting blood transfusions now, just to push her numbers up for the blood test tomorrow and boost her for the chemo treatment on Thursday. The infection was in her throat and went down into the esophagus causing heartburn. The doctor said the infection was unusual. She will be sent home with an antibiotic; she's still on her Stryker Sleep Number bed — aaahhhh! She hopes to be out of there to get to

RPCI by 8:30 a.m. tomorrow. She will drive her father's car to RPCI.

4/12-14/11 - Chemo Procedure: Andriamycin.

4/19/11, Tues. —

Charron at RPCI called that Debra is scheduled to see Dr. LaiLai after her blood test; and the MUGA test on her heart; didn't know results; get to the hospital and knock it out of the park; 50,000 platelets; the hospital will send records and the blood test to Dr. LaiLai.

4/21/11, Thurs. —

Debra had her last chemo treatment today, (*God willing*). They didn't say it was her last one, but another old lady "graduated" from her treatments and the nurses played the music for graduation, put a graduation cap on her, clapped and said she has graduated. She was so surprised! Deb asked the nurses how did the woman know she is clear. The nurses said through a CT scan, but they brought her in for another treatment? Debra was confused. "Mom, will the nurses do that for me? I hope you're here, Mommy, but it would be the best present I can give Jeremy." "Whenever, it is, Debra, it will be such an achievement for you. You've gone through a lot and have taken everything they have given you like a trooper. You have shown such strength that I, frankly, never knew you had. You were always my Princess! (*Labels on clothing bothered her, chair pads, wash cloths, some materials, you name it.*) We laughed and laughed. 👍👍 "See, Mom, there was a reason why we couldn't go to Florida. God had His own plan for me."

Upstate delivers Emend 125-80 mg, Dexamethasone 4 mg, Omeprazole DR 20 mg.

4/29/11, Fri. —

Personal: She's still at Lisa's, everybody at Chris' house is sick with sore throats. She and Lisa are sitting outside, it's 60! "We were going to do gardening but with all the rain, the yard is soaking and flooded." She's getting a lot of sleep. Lisa has a sunroom at front of house with a cot and TV and she sleeps there. Lisa has her own medical problems; takes a lot of medicine.

"Mom, for your anniversary, are you going back to your island? Is Boldt Castle still being fixed?" (*If we can manage it what with our NYC trip, Ellis Island, NYC, Empire State Building. And Jerr and I were married at Boldt Castle in the Thousand Islands.*)

Personal: Donna will probably get her truck back on the road; she's fixing her muffler for $180. We're clearing out grandma's clothes (after ten years).

No news about her Disability claim yet; she dropped off her papers on 4/15, but the representative said, "Oh sure, no problem." But how long does it take? She also said she doesn't know the reason she's keeping all her stuff in Chris' attic because when she gets her own apartment again, she will save all the money she gets and will buy all new furniture again. Jeremy deserves new furniture again in a good apartment. "But, Mom, when you have time, we'll go through all the stuff, and decide if it's worth keeping. Some mementoes that mean a lot to me, I will keep."

5/2/11, Mon. —

Debra had her blood test before going for a CT scan at RPCI, but she said she's very weak and breathless, she feels like she has the weight of the world on her shoulders, like a huge board across her shoulders and her mid-back hurts. Maybe it is from all the rain. She's prepared in case they tell her she has to continue chemo-therapy. ⚲ She has another tooth infection and a huge abscess. Chemo affects the whole body. Her throat hurts; she's taking antibiotics again. She has a vague tingling in her feet but not in her hands this time; she was told she could have permanent nerve damage. Having injections at Buffalo and a 24 minute MUGA test/heart/could affect heart/injection; there's big screen over you. At RPCI, was told her blood was OK; then went to the 3rd Floor for MUGA test; back down to the 2nd Floor for EKG. "Mom, I waited 1-½ hours, saw doctor for one minute; he was in and out of the room before I could blink." The muscles in her stomach hurt; she drinks a case of water. "Mummy, I am prepared in case RPCI tell me I have to continue with chemo. I don't know why after two other hospitals tell me I'm clear that RPCI tell me I'm not! I have another tooth infection, a huge abscess which hurts my throat; I need antibiotics. Why is this popping up now; does chemo affect your gums and teeth?" She is looking forward to getting her teeth done and maybe getting an implant for the missing teeth.

Personal: "Outside, it's 14°; it snowed most of week. Donna's company is sponsoring a marathon on 5/20 for cancer at Hyde Park; she put in $5 for you, Mom."

Personal: "Donna is getting better. (*Thank, God.*) We went to Save-a-Lot and bought her loads of groceries and a case of water. I carried the bags upstairs for her, since the muscles in her stomach are painful. She has lunch with Jim once a week. DJ, her friend from Vancouver, is here to visit his parents."

5/3/11, Tues. —

While we were talking today, Charron at RPCI was trying to reach Debra. She is to go to the E/R immediately! Her blood count is so low, she needs blood! Charron will call the hospital to expect her — now!

Debra: "I feel worse today, Mom, can hardly breathe. I can't even dress; I'm going to go to the hospital in my pajamas. I can barely lift the phone. Chris is coming home to take me. You'll never be able to get here in time, please. Charron said I feel that way because there's no blood circulating in my body."

Immediately, when Debra arrived at the E/R, she was started on a blood transfusion. The nurses could not find a vein; they tried and tried; finally went up under her arm near her armpit. She screamed in pain. (*Months later, she still had a baseball-sized black bruise under her armpit.*)

Debra's blood count was **6** and the doctor said she could have gone into cardiac arrest! She received five pints of blood and four bags of platelets, and a pain shot for something; she can't remember. She was finally admitted. She was crying. "Where does the blood go; why do I have to keep doing this?" She was told the platelets have to build up. Usually she was told they don't do blood transfusions in the E/R. When the E/R nurse came in, Debra mentioned she hadn't eaten all day; she was there for three hours and still had not received a tray of food. Then in ten minutes, she had a tray of goulash heated up and sandwiches. "Yum, Mommy, there's angels all around me."

She has an appointment with her pain management doctor on 5/17. (*This is not the pain management doctor associated with RPCI.*) " I don't want to miss that appointment. She is so wonderful and helps me a lot, even when she to give me the injections into my back." (*We told her we'd take her no matter what, unless she was in the hospital again.*)

5/4/11, Wed. —

Another blood test today; she saw a different doctor, 1-½ low platelets. On Monday, Debra talked about the dentist before she goes in. She feels great; no pain! *Hallelujah!* She was informed she'll have a CT scan in three weeks in Buffalo. Her thumb nails hurt. She can't afford to be low on protein.

Personal: She stayed at Lisa's; she took her Jeep downtown. Painted her bathroom for her; a real nice tan since her woodwork is brown. It looks so nice.

5/8/11, Sun., Mother's Day. —

Debra called me "HAPPY MOTHER'S DAY, MUMMY". She was all chipper and happy and said, "Mummy, I'm home!" I called her the bionic woman. She said, "Or a vampire?" We were laughing. I told her Happy Mother's Day to you, sweetheart. She said, "Becoming a mother was the best gift I ever had; Jeremy was just a beautiful baby, and he's growing to be a wonderful young man. I just hope I can continue to guide him in the right thing to do." *(He was a beautiful baby because you are a beautiful person. He has your long eyelashes and beautiful skin and a sweet disposition — but he's very strong-willed. Hmmm, does that sound familiar?)* ⚓ ⚓ "You know, Mom, Jeremy should have a proper home, a loving, nurturing home, where he is loved to the skies. I'm going to make sure he gets that home. He knows I love him so much, and I want to once again provide a home where he's free to express his feelings, to play on his games, to be outside in the woods, to do whatever makes him happy — that's what this Mother — me — wants for him. One day...... *"And we'll help you to do that again, Debra."*

Later, Debra called me and immediately said, "Mom, I'm sorry I didn't get your card in the mail to you, but this is what my card says. As she read it, and I heard her voice and words in my ear, I was crying.

5/9/11, Mon. —

Upstate delivers Dexamethasone 4 mg.

5/10/11, Tues. —

Debra went for CT scan; she sees Dr. LaiLai on Thursday.

5/11/11, Wed. —

After Debra sees Dr. LaiLai, Lisa has to take her mother for her mammogram. Her mother has had her last chemo treatment and was cleared of her cancer. They were watching a cyst in her kidney which was benign. She was given a powder for her scalp so that her thinning hair doesn't show as much, Lisa said.

Personal: Jeremy gave Debra a card and a dozen roses. Chris usually gives her a card, too. She is working on Lisa's garden, used natural stones, painted their living room and Lisa's other bathroom. It has been 10 years. They have a big yard goes back almost to Oppenheim Zoo, they see deer and squirrels, of course. Jeremy, who goes hunting with his father, got a deer this year but not a buck. *"Grandma was sick about this thought!"* He is 15 years old this year. Ginny has been invited to her sister's. She is redoing her kitchen with cherry cabinets and wood floors. She then said "When Chris moves in, it will all be done." ("What did she just say to me, Mom?!") *Debra said "I certainly hope he is no longer working then because in addition to the hour he has to drive to work at 5:00 in the morning, her house is yet another 30 minutes in the opposite direction!"*

5/12/11, Thurs. — CT Scan performed.

Dr. LaiLai actually spent a few minutes with her; said the cancer is not gone; but it has diminished considerably.

Debra asked: Can you explain to me why it is just a little spot and doesn't go away?

Dr. LaiLai: It is one cell comprised of 10 or 20 cells that make up the tiny spot. Before it was a cluster of 40-60 cells. I can't put a measurement on it; it's like the dot of an i.

Debra: "What happens to all the blood? Why do I keep having to have blood transfusions?"

Dr. LaiLai: The body can't replenish it, your body uses it all; I'm not worried but I don't want to wait to start chemo again.

Debra was scheduled for next Thursday.

Dr. LaiLai is going to insert a port in her chest saying it's no big deal, just a tiny incision, and blood will be able to be taken via the port (an implantable vascular access port*), and she will be able to have her chemo administered there, too. (*In 2009 at the beginning of her treatments when the doctor initially mentioned the port to Debra, she said it sounded so gross to her, and she did not want an apparatus sticking out of her chest or wherever they put it. It was never brought up again.*)

Now, she stated "I will accept this, I don't want to be stuck 6-10 times just for them to get blood; it hurts too much. I scream and cry. So I'll be able to stay with you this summer for my next three treatments, is my room still there, Mummy?"

(*Of course, sweetheart, always! But let me ask you, the doctor is going to insert it into your right breast? Would the insertion of this port be any more painful than the rose tattoo you had done on your left breast? You've told me the horrible story about how Phil had it done, and I was not happy about it at the time, either with you or Phil. I cried and cried about the destruction of your beautiful skin. At least this will be done in a hospital under sedation!*) (*Now I get a small smile from Debra, "I guess not more painful, Mom."*)

5/17/11 - Phlebotomy Unit for blood work.

5/18/11

Upstate delivers Emend 125-80 mg, Omeprazole DR 20 mg.

5/20/11, Fri. — Chemo Procedure: Cisplatin. MUGA test to evaluate for Adriamycin. Stayed at Lisa's.

5/20/11, Fri. —

Donna, through her work as Activities Director of a nursing home, organized participants at "Inspiration" by the American Cancer Society, a relay race, from 3:30-10:30, 15 people on a team and somebody has to be on the track at all times. Debra and Jeremy participated, it was held at a stadium in Niagara Falls. Debra made one full circle; Jeremy wanted to continue, but she couldn't.

5/22/11, Sun. — Enroute from Florida.

Jerr and I stopped at the Grove City Outlet Mall and after lunch at Eat 'N Park, we shopped — went to Anne Loft and purchased tops for the girls, then to Old Navy and a few other stops.

5/23/11, Mon. —

Debra had the port inserted but had a bad reaction from it. She didn't feel anything during the procedure but wasn't aware of anything for three days! Lisa said she could talk but she said she wasn't aware of what she was saying. Then she got severe pain in her knees, like somebody had hit her with a bat.

5/30/11, Mon. — @ NFMMH —

Donna took Debra to the hospital at 1:00 a.m. Debra's throat was swollen up and she couldn't talk or swallow. Doctors found that she had an infection in her throat and a yeast infection; started her on IVs and antibiotics. She was started on blood and platelets again and pain shots for pain in her chest (*Are the shingles* back?)

6/1/11, Wed. — (Our anniversary) —

Debra placed a wrenching phone message at our home that she was in NFMMH and wanted to see us — please, Mommy! When we heard the message, Jerr and I immediately left for Niagara Falls. We stopped at the dairy store because Jerr wanted to take her a huge strawberry milk shake. She loved it!

When she had called us earlier, she had been in such pain and was so scared, but she told us she was so grateful that she had the port installed because all needles were going in there and it was no problem now, no pain. She still had baseball-sized bruises on her arms and under her armpits from her last hospital stay a month ago where the nurses couldn't even find the veins any more and the needles were really hurting her. (*Lisa informed us that once when she took Debra to the E/R, she had to be injected* **eight** *times before a nurse(s) found a vein — one under her armpit! Debra was screaming in pain.*)

"Mom, why didn't I have this port done before?! Why did no one bring the subject of the port up again? Why? Why? Didn't the nurses report the problems with the needles? Did they think I enjoyed the needles and the pain? Why couldn't someone some- where just sit for a few minutes and explain it to me again — or to us" All we could do was hold her and hug her and kiss her — her lips tasted of strawberry milk shake! 🛆 🛆 It was about 7:00 p.m. when she fell asleep, so peaceful now. We stayed another hour and left to return home.

Personal: Jerr and I stopped at the Como at the Airport Restaurant for dinner. The waitress overheard Jerr and me toasting each other with water, "Well....happy anniversary, sweetheart." She told our friend, Frank, the owner who sent over wine and beer. When we went to check out, we were told he had picked up the entire dinner tab, and as we were leaving and hugging him and saying "thank you and goodbye", he gave us two large pizza breads (*they are the best!*). His mother, Adeline, was feeling under the weather and didn't come in that day but he called her and told her we were there. She said, they better come back to see me, or else......"

Later that evening, we kept calling Debra and there was no answer. As usual, she had left her charger at her father's house, and he kept saying it wasn't there, that it was at Lisa's. What a pathetic trick and what to do to her in her pain. When we were finally able to talk to her, we told her about Como's and she sounded like she was smiling and said, "See, Mom, angels are all around you, too."

6/3/11, Fri. — @ NFMMH. —

On our way to Niagara Falls, Jerr wanted to stop at the famous Ted's Hot Dogs because Debra said she was yearning for one; she was so hungry. So here we go into her hospital room with the aroma of Ted's hot dogs, relish, fries, the ketchup she loves and an ice cold drink. We were there when doctor came in to see her and said her counts were up but only to 30,000; (normal is 100,000); they would like to see them higher, but she could probably go home Saturday. The doctor smiled and said, "Boy, is there a delicious aroma in here!" 🔼

6/5/11, Sun. —

Erma's email was that their local Relay for Life was held on Friday, 6/3/11 and Debra's name was announced during the *luminaria* ceremony. (*Dear, God, thank you for family or people who have the empathy for others in their difficult situation, but did they have to endure the pain they did in order to do Your work?*)

6/6/11, Mon. —

Debra discharged from NFMMH with instructions to follow-up with Dr. LaiLai by 6/7/11, blood work 6/8/11, and what to watch for — chest pain, shortness of breath, nausea, vomiting, or diarrhea.

She's been given a prescription for needles to inject in her stomach to build up her blood. (*What?!*) She teased Jerr that she was doing what he was doing with his insulin shots! *My, God, sweetheart, I hope not! You don't want to keep doing this! But shots in your stomach?"* "Well, Jerr, the doctor said it was only temporary, so we'll see." (*I have always had such a phobia about needles, I felt weak in the knees and had to sit down at the thought of my little girl injecting herself — OMG. I can't even look at Jerr doing it.*)

6/8/11

Upstate delivers Emend 125-80 mg.

6/9/11, Thurs. — Chemo Procedure: Cisplatin. MUGA test to evaluation for Adriamycin.

After Debra's chemo treatment, we stopped at the Cracker Barrel for "lundin."

6/10/11, Fri —

Actually, today we had dinner at home. We were all tired from the five hour stay at the Amherst Clinic.

6/11/11, Sat. —

Debra still with us but on the way home, we stopped for a Mexican restaurant in Town of Tonawanda — El Palenque Grill, which Debra recommende; she and Chris had found it. Fabulous!

6/12/11, Sun. — St. Gregory Church and it was like finally coming home.

6/17/11, Fri. —

When we returned home from Debra's chemo treatment; she wanted to go to Spoth's Garden Shop to get Jerr's Father's Day present surprise. Then we stopped to buy landscape lights to outline the curves of the garden. She immediately planted the flowers and installed the lights and called him outside to see his surprise. She made him promise to go outside in the evening and see how everything looks! Her card read: Of all the men I know, you are the perfect example of a father's love.

(The garden was beautiful. And before she left, we hugged her, said "thank you, and I love you." She answered "I love you two, too. And a group hug. And, yes, that evening, we enjoyed the lights.") 🕯️🕯️

Donna's card included a "I'M THE BOSS" button and read, "Dad, on

Father's Day, wear this button to show your position of authority in the family! But...don't forget to give it back to Mom tomorrow!"

Personal: Debra tells us the story that after another one of Debra's chemo treatments, she and Lisa were starved and they stopped at Country Style Buffet. They ate and ate; Debra said probably from nerves but then she always feels starved after her treatments. When they got home, the boys said they were hungry and asked what was for dinner. Debra and Lisa looked at each other — oh, yuk! 👍 👍

6/28/11, Tues. —

Debra's BIRTHDAY! She didn't want to do anything today. "Happy birthday, my little Princess!"

She was beginning to feel sick and called RPCI, Dr. LaiLai's office. She was told she needed to have her blood tests done first. So on Wednesday afternoon had a blood test and was told the results were low. She left there and tried getting into NFMMH, who said they had no room. She called Dr. LaiLai's office again and was told to go to the Amherst clinic, so back she goes for another blood test and Yvonne started her on platelets and then she was rushed out and sent home. We were to remember this date!

Upstate delivers Emend 125-80 mg, Omeprazole DR 20 mg.

6/29/11, Wed. —

Debra went to NFMMH for more blood tests. (*We had gone to The Viking Shop and bought a garden plaque for her birthday. She loved it.*)

Upstate delivers Dexamethasone 4 mg.

6/30/11, Thurs. — @ E/R MSMH

When the results of Debra's blood tests came in, her blood count was **6!** She was immediately admitted. When her eyelids were pulled down it showed she was super anemic. There were white spots in her throat from an infection.

7/1/11, Fri., 1:00 p.m. @ MSMH —

Jerr and I went to Lewiston to see Debra, stopping en route to Lewiston so Jerr could buy Debra a Wild Berry Yoghurt Parfait from Wendy's on Grand Island. We asked for a large cup of ice (to keep it cold).

Debra was in Room 303, the sign on the floor read, "Cardiac/Pulmonary Floor (*What?*) Before we entered Debra's room, there was another sign that all visitors had to wear masks and coats! What was this about? (*We looked like space aliens in the yellow coats but learned from Debra this was to stop the danger of infection.*)

As we were asking why she was on a cardiac floor, the cardiologist came in and told her there was tissue damage to her heart because of the low blood count and that the damage was recent. He told us, "Tissue dies where there is no blood. When did you have your last blood test?"

Debra told him that on 6/28 she had gone to RPCI's Amherst Clinic and given platelets and told she was OK and sent home. She had reported to the nurses that she had a pain in the middle of her back that was unlike the pain she had with shingles.

The cardiologist stated that she had probably had a mild heart attack! He said in view of the more serious issues she had, there probably wasn't a treatment protocol that he could suggest at this time. When she was finished with her chemo, she could pursue the heart problem with him. She has had a heart murmur. She had been up all night and couldn't sleep and was very uncomfortable.

Personal: Later, before Jerr and I left the hospital, we discussed where we could stop for dinner, but it was late, we did NOT want to stop anywhere in Niagara Falls, the Como was closed, so we stopped at Tim Horton's in the hospital for a small snack.

Debra receives Spiritual Care.

Personal: Talked to Donna, told her Debra was in hospital. Donna said she's going with her other friend, Lisa, to Varysburg for a 4th of July concert; she's driving her own car since she wants to come home as she's working on Tuesday and Lisa is remaining there.

7/2/11, Sat., 10:00 a.m. @ MSMH —

A different cardiologist came in and confirmed that Debra had tissue damage to her heart because of low blood and that it was recent damage. Deb again told about her the 6/28 incident.

She also found out that there were options as to where the port was inserted; it did not have to be front and center in her chest! Neither Dr. LaiLai nor Charron informed her about any side effects from the surgery to insert the port. The cardiologist will see Debra again when he has the results from the morning's blood work. The tissue problem in her heart doesn't affect how the heart functions. He told her she can have chemo at a clinic where Lisa took her mother near Summit Mall in Niagara Falls (*not RPCI!*). Lisa told me she didn't like RPCI either or how some of the staff treated Debra. (*And why? Debra has always been so sweet to people until she reaches her limit and is in pain.*)

7/3/11, Sun. @ MSMH —

Doctor said that today her count is 2 and the doctor wants it to be at least 4 before he lets her go home. She's being given Neupragin* shots which raise her white blood cells in the bone marrow. She's still being given an antibiotic. Dr. Heshin (?) saw her today. The nausea is OK; she likes Boost or Walgreen's chocolate energy drink; some of the others have a lot of sodium, and she doesn't like them. She had eggs and toast for breakfast. She has been eating and having regular bowel movements. Today her male nurse told her a joke about a very religious woman and her two pigeons. They were laughing and laughing. 🕊️🕊️ (*It was a funny joke.*)

Personal: Lisa and Doug stopped at the hospital on their way from Old Fort Niagara and dropped off her phone charger.

8:30 p.m. —

Debra has been nauseated, didn't eat lunch or dinner; she was hungry but when she smelled the food, she couldn't eat it. She was given something for the nausea; she'll ask for something light later on — a yoghurt, Jell-O, or ice cream. Doctor hasn't come back so she'll probably see him tomorrow. She has been on a heart monitor. Gave us the phone number to her room.

7/4/11, Mon. - 4th of July @ MSMH -Debra's call

From her room, she can see the fireworks from a couple of communities. "Mom, do you remember when we used to go the river for fireworks? You had found a great spot again and it was a beautiful night, then Jerr took me and Chris to dinner at the Olympic Restaurant and it was 11:00 p.m.? My goodness, it was after 1:00 a.m. and you said it was the latest you had been out forever!" We were laughing. 🛏️🛏️

Debra receives Spiritual Care today.

7/5/11, Tues. @ MSMH —

The doctor is going to keep monitoring how her body is responding to the oral antibiotics vs. the IV ones and then discharge her. Her blood levels must be OK.....BUT that she has conjunctivitis in her eye! She thought all night that she had something in her eye, or that she had been bitten by a bug or spider (In the hospital?), and her eye was gummed shut this morning. The doctor is giving her a special eye drop to clear it up. *Doesn't the attack on her body ever stop?*

Later, she said she feels like she has a cold, keeps clearing her throat; blood tests looks good; she called Charron for a copy of the blood tests when she went to Amherst on 6/28/11. (**Never received them.**)

Today, Debra receives Spiritual Care.

7/6/11, Wed. @ MSMH —

Debra said not to come to the hospital today; she was probably going to be discharged and later, learned she was discharged at 7:30 p.m.

7/7/11, Thurs. — Chemo Procedure of Cisplatin cancelled. MUGA test to evaluation for Adriamycin postponed.

7/7/11, Thurs., 9:30 p.m. @ MSMH —

Debra's has been sleeping most of the day; she still doesn't feel well, she's winded, breathless, doctor told her to get rest, and she feels wiped out. The doctor also asked why she isn't getting the shots to build up her red blood cells in her bone marrow?! He said she needs to tell Dr. LaiLai that she needs the shots! (*What shots? Are these the same shots she's been giving in her stomach? Why should she have to ask — LaiLai and others are the experts, aren't they? What do we know?!*)

7/8/11, Fri. @ MSMH —

Debra has been given two bags of platelets and four blood transfusions. She has pain in her back and severe pain in her head. She said she thought she was going to be told she has a brain tumor and die, it was so bad. There are only 15 pints of blood in body; did her count of 4 mean she only had 4 pints of blood left?

7/12/11, Tues., 7:30 p.m. @ MSMH —

Debra has been sleeping most of the day.

Personal: The other day while Debra and Lisa had gone to a store, Colton had gone to the DMV across the street, and he locked the car door, and they couldn't get back in because it has a special anti-theft lock. It was so, so hot and there was no shade. Debra was sitting on the curb. She looked so bad, Lisa wanted to take her to the hospital. They called Chris who came and dismantled the door and the lock, and they were able to get in.

Later during the middle of the night, she felt she needed to go to MSMH to have her blood checked. The E/R was packed, but they ran a pure vein blood enzyme test and all readings were OK. The doctor told her the antibiotics were still working in her body and that's probably why she felt like she had a flu or cold. Her nose is drippy and her shoulders ache, and she still has the pain in her back. The doctor said it would probably be a year after the end of chemo before her body would be back to normal. Chris has no air conditioning in his house although he's redoing all the ducts to put in a new air conditioner. She just can't take the heat right now. She's still at Lisa's.

Personal: Donna is feeling better; she has been sick. Jeremy and Debra are coming to maybe swim or go to Lasertron. She doesn't know if she will feel like being anywhere. She said it was too hot to go to Old Home Days here in Williamsville. I informed her that we're taking Mark to Buffalo for his own chemo treatment, but they could come over anyway, and she said that's OK.

7/16/11, Sat., 6:30 p.m. —

Debra and Jeremy want to come swimming tomorrow, Sunday, and then we will drive Jeremy home to Buffalo.

I go to church from 11:00 to 12:30 so I could meet her if Lisa drops her off at the halfway point. Debra is still feeling tired but wants to go through the chemo treatment on Thursday. She still has not received the blood test report she requested; the one on 6/28/11. She's also going to request the last three MUGA tests. They have to use an IV in a vein for a pure sample and not through the port. She recalls all the painful needles all over again.

Spent the whole afternoon at the pool. Debra and Jeremy in the water, talking and talking and laughing. Then when they came out for a bit, she checked his shoulders and sprays some more sun screen on him.

7/20/11, Wed. —

Debra called RPCI, (Charron) and said she wanted to change her chemo appointment for next Thursday, 7/28, because everybody was out of town; she had no car and no one to give her a ride and there's no one available to care for her if she has to go to the hospital as usual.

Personal: Jeremy got out of orientation today and he's spending the rest of the week and week-end with Debra. "What a happy time", she said. Lisa and Doug are going to Rochester, so Chris is coming over, and they are going to BBQ and have time together -- in the quiet, peaceful neighborhood. Hopefully, before the weekend, Chris will finally take her to get her new phone — her birthday present! With her numb fingertips, she's had trouble dialing on the tiny buttons on this phone.

8/3/11, Wed.

After Debra's appointment, we stopped for "lundin" again at the Anchor Bar.

8/4/11

Upstate delivers Omeprazole DR 20 mg.

8/3/11, Wed. — Blood work at RPCI. We left message asking how things had gone.

8/4/11, Thurs. — CT Scan of chest, abdomen, pelvis.

8/5/11, Fri. — Appointment with Dr. LaiLai in Amherst.

8/9/11, Tues., 11:40 a.m. —

Debra didn't go for the CT scan because it was scheduled at 7:00 a.m. and it was a fasting test. She just couldn't hold off without food, she was dizzy; besides she had a cold (probably from air conditioning last week when it was so hot). When she went outside, she felt like just falling down, the sun was so hot; she also thought it was low blood chemistry, but she recovered.

8/12/11, Fri. 1:00 p.m. —

The CT scan was rescheduled for today. Lisa is taking her. Then for her conference meeting with Dr. LaiLai is on 8/25 and we're taking her. She doesn't remember the time. Chris is coming over on Friday. (*Does that take care of the weekend?*)

Told her the Lewiston Art Festival is this weekend and that we're going — weather depending.

Then we talked about the Erie County Fair and that everybody wants to go. We always take them, but if it is too hot, let's rethink this. "No, we want to go, Mom. We always go. I want to keep things normal."

"Mom, speaking about the fairs and craft shows, do you remember the 'memory boxes' you made Jeremy? You are such a master recycler! You saved everything from items which are usually thrown away — plastic bits, plastic ties, the pizza stands so the lid doesn't get crushed, pop caps, everything. We would sit days and you made Jeremy memory boxes. It was so awesome how you made all the saved bits and pieces come to life as furniture, tables, fireplaces, rugs, picture frames, whatever. And when your friends found out about them, they had you make them for their children." (*I made "memory boxes" out of a clear plastic shoe box, laid it sideways and created a scene of a child's favorite places or room or hobby. Jeremy's first 'memory box' was a log cabin — I cut out wildlife pictures from catalogues and magazines, evergreens, a rug, furniture, sleeping cot, then outside was a campfire, logs, real branches from our pine trees. When we finished, all you had to do was put the lid on, and it was stacked away.*)

"Deb, do you remember when friends brought samples of their

kids' wallpaper or favorite colors or hobbies, and one night, I knocked the box over and couldn't remember whose wallpaper was whose — was it Lucy's, or Jilies, or Kelly's or Matt's or Jimmy's — we sorted it out eventually and everything got put into its proper place and in time for a special event for them!! You even offered to go investigate the kids' rooms and make notes about their wallpaper!"

8/11/11, Thurs. — Chemo Procedure: Cisplatin.

8/19/11, Fri., 8:30 p.m. —

The Wheatfield Festival is this weekend and Debra and Jeremy will go there instead of the Erie County Fair because of the distance for them. Jeremy's friend's father has a gun table at the Fair, and he has received four passes and three other friends are going to get in.

Also, this weekend is Scottish Festival, which we will go to at Tonawanda Creek.

When Debra had her CT scan, she came home to take a little nap and the next thing she knew Lisa was telling her it was 4:30 p.m. She had forgotten how it affected her. (*Isn't Ambien for blocked arteries?*)

Personal: "Mom, my idea about having "Bulldog Boards" (skateboards) is gone! My feelings are hurt." She went on to tell me several other issues that someone else was doing and events that have hurt her and asks how people can hurt her so much? (crying)

"Debra, I can understand how you feel. But all those things are material things, they are not important in the long run. And then maybe none of their plans will materialize. You are getting yourself all upset when you shouldn't. But perhaps talk to her about it — when you see her. Maybe it's a misunderstanding."

"But, Mom, feelings are forever."

"Yes, that's why you should be in a positive environment and let's think good thoughts. When your plans materialize, we'll help you. With one condition, I want your first skateboard signed, and I want it called "Mama Bulldog!" 🛹🛹

"Mom, Chris and I had a long 3-hour talk; we sat in the car outside Lisa's house. He said, "You're not coming back home, are you, Deb?"

Debra: "Look around here, Chris, from every window I see a beautiful view; there's a quiet street, peaceful woods, it's quiet; there are three kids next door on one side and four kids on the other side and you don't hear them. It's truly peaceful here."

Debra talked to the lawyer, who said she has to apply for Social Security first and then when she hears from them whether it's an approval or rejection, then he can do something. If Social Security declines her, then he will jump in and help. "We'll apply for other money", he said. She can't get compensation because that's job-related, but they have 30 days to respond.

8/19/11, Fri. — CT scan performed. Lisa took Debra to Buffalo.

8/25/11, Thurs., 2:00 p.m. @ RPCI, Amherst Center — Appointment with Dr. LaiLai.

Dr. LaiLai did not see her/us until 3:30 p.m. at the Amherst Clinic; we were the last ones there and had been there since 1:00 p.m. Nor would anyone tell us what was going on. Finally, Debra was examined internally by Dr. LaiLai. Then one of the secretaries came to waiting room to get me and told me I could sit in the conference room.

Dr. LaiLai stood in the doorway and said, "Wait here. We're admitting Debra to the hospital on Monday.

Lorr: Why?

Dr.:   It's gotten worse.

Lorr: What happened? *I was stunned.*

Dr.:   Charron will come and talk to you." He then turned around and went down the hallway.

When Charron came in, she said Debra would have to be admitted for the next treatment because of the serious side effects of the chemo. It would be a one-hour treatment on the 1st day and then a 12-hour treatment. She could become disoriented and have hallucinations, and they wouldn't want her doing anything "rash".

Lorr: What has Debra said?

Charron: She signed for the treatment.

Lorr: We couldn't understand why the doctor waited until now to do this when the other treatment didn't seem to be working. (Did not get an answer.)

Lisa came back to the conference room because she was concerned I was taking so long. We talked about why this couldn't be treated by surgery?

Charron: Every cancer is different and no two are alike and no treatment is the same, but we could talk to the doctor.

Lorr: When? He didn't have time to talk to me now.

Charron: He talked to Debra. She signed for the treatment.

Lorr: I would like to speak to Dr. LaiLai again with Debra.

Lisa: Dr. LaiLai? He has left the Office, we saw him leave when we were in the waiting room!

We again asked for the report of the first CT scan and the last one and the copy of the blood test of 6/28/11. She wrote down a phone number for us to get this information. She said it was their office.

Lorr: (*WHY??? Why couldn't she get this for Debra???*)

When Dr. LaiLai told Debra the results of the CT Scan, he said "It's not stronger; it's different."

"Mom, I don't want you to go to bed upset tonight."

"Sweetheart, neither do I want you to be upset. Do you want to talk about it?"

"No, Mom, it is what it is. Obviously, I can't change it."

"Oh, by the way, I have a phone interview with Social Security at 9:00 a.m. on Monday. The last time I looked at my statement, I will get $859!"

(*We stopped at Perkins Restaurant for dinner — a very quiet one, each one of us deep in thought.*)

8/28/11, Sun. —

At St. Gregory's today, my spirit was numb, my prayers were routine, my petitions just wouldn't come out. Why? I left the church and came home.

Debra has a 9:00 a.m. phone interview with Social Security tomorrow, Mon., 8/29/11. She has all the information in front of her, dates, phone numbers for doctors, hospitals, etc. She's ready to answer any of their questions.

She will give RPCI until 11:00 a.m. to call her and then she will call them.

Lisa will drop her off at the usual place on Niagara Falls Blvd & Robinson in North Tonawanda. We will pick Debra up and take her the rest of the way to Buffalo. I told her Jerr and I will stay with her at RPCI for the three days even if we have to sleep in the waiting room, but we're not leaving her alone any more. I packed a bag for us.

8/29, 30, 31/11 - Chemo Procedure: Ifosfamide*.

8/29/11, Mon. —

Debra had her 1-½ hour telephone interview with Social Security. The rep said their investigation may go back to 2009 when she was first diagnosed. (Angels, Mom!)

During her interview, Charron from RPCI called that Debra had to check into the hospital, and we took her. She was hungry so we stopped at Tim Horton's for lunch and then went directly to the hospital.

Deb was admitted at 1:30 p.m. to Room #6409, 6 West. Her nurses were Debi and Diane. She had asked for pain meds, and she finally got Dilaudid at 4:30 p.m. She had severe pain in her legs up the shin bone to her knee, her hands were numb past her wrist, and she had severe pain in the left back. She has had that pain for 25 hours, she felt she slept wrong or twisted it somehow.

This hospital is so much better than being in Amherst; it's such a relief, they are catering to her, she's right now in a private room, and not with old, very sick people, gagging like at Amherst, and the nurses are quietly laughing and joking with each other in the center station.

Jerr and I went to the Waiting Room on the 6th Floor, when we came back, the two nurses at the station asked how we were doing. I asked about the procedure — the 1-hour chemo and then the 12-hour chemo and the horrible side effects. I told them that we are going to spend the nights in the waiting room because of the 'side effects' — that we didn't want Debra to be alone. "We want to be with her and that she knows that we are with her."

They looked at each other puzzled, and Diane said, "What side effects?" I told her we were told there would be serious side affects. I told them what we had been told.

Diane: Who told you that?

L: Charron.

They looked at each other again and said Charron..?

L: Yes.

And one of them just huffed and they didn't say anything.

Then they said the chemo would be given at the same time and there shouldn't **be** any side effects. We were welcome to stay if we wanted to, but it really wasn't necessary; Debra would be closely monitored.

5:30 p.m.

Dr. Frederick and Dr. Godoy came to see her. They must have been informed that we were questioning the procedure. They said, the reason she was admitted to RPCI was to monitor her bladder since Ifosfamide might cause bladder bleeding, and if it did, they can address it immediately. It was Dr. Godoy who ordered the pain meds, and she said she'd be back to see Debra tomorrow. I asked about the side effects of this chemo and they said there shouldn't be any! (*Angels, or God's intervention, thank you, God! Thank You.*)

We stayed with Debra until 9:00 p.m., and she was sleeping most of the time. She called us later:

"Mom, my room may be a Godsend. Through the windows, I can see the skyline of Buffalo, the lights are beautiful, and I can see down the entire street, it looks like a runway. Then in the distance is the Niagara river — so quiet, so beautiful."

Bess, her evening nurse, gave her chocolate pudding. She had her pain shot ready without argument, no Amend, no nausea, Prilosec was OK when she was given it for stomach pain, and she dreaded going back to the Amherst Clinic. "Mom, I never told you, but I HATE, HATE, HATED IT!!! I was so anxious every time I had to go there, had to sit next to some fairly young guy gagging and choking to death with lung cancer; seeing everybody else so down and sick; there was no privacy and all the chaos of the nurse's station, you know noise makes me anxious and nervous. And here, this is so relaxing."

(I never knew her feeling about Amherst; she always seemed so positive and smiling at everybody there and thanking them for the smallest kindnesses. I didn't say anything and tried to stay positive, too. She had initially agreed to go to the Amherst Clinic because of the two mile distance from our house vs. the distance to downtown Buffalo.

8/30/11, Tues., 10:30 a.m. —

We were on our way to Buffalo when Debra called and said she had a wonderful night, was finally able to sleep, her bladder is clear with no bleeding! (*Thank God!*) She was started on the second course of Ifosfamide at 4:30 p.m. together with Mesna*. She was off the hose all day, given a scented bath wash/shampoo, and she feels like Ivana Trump at the spa!

She was given Purell antibiotic hand wash — the kind you pay $2 or $3 in the drugstore. She's going to give herself a Mary Kay mask and facial that I gave her for her birthday, products she's used forever. (As a matter of fact, the three of us had been chosen for a professional photo shoot in "Women of Mary Kay." That photo is my favorite one.)

For breakfast, she thought she would get a bagel and juice, but when she lifted the cover, "There was scrambled eggs, pancakes, mandarin oranges 'Mom, drained just like I like them!', toast, sausage patty, milk, banana bread, Boost, cranberry which I didn't drink because it makes my throat dry. Wow! Mom, there are angels around me. At MSMH, it has the worse food, then NFMMH, then the best ones are Suburban and RPCI." She said, "Take your time getting here; I'm OK now!" I asked, "Are you sure you aren't going to the hospitals just for the food?!" "Yeah, sure, Mom!" 🛅 🛅

We got to Buffalo about 3:30 and at 3:45 p.m., Bess came in with a trainee and they started Debra's Mesna and then 15 min. later, the Ifosfamide. Dr. LaiLai came in with Dr. Goody and asked how Debra was and that she would be discharged tomorrow. He wouldn't talk to Jerr or me. At 5:30 p.m., her dinner came, she was able to manage her own dinner. Later, Jerr and I stopped for our own dinner on the way home.

8/31/11, Wed., 9:30 a.m. —

Nurse: Sandi and HCA Candi. Doctors came in, they are going to keep her another day because of her spasms in her arms; from her elbows to her thumbs; she can't control her movements (like a person with Parkinson's disease, she said). They stopped giving her the chemo and the sodium chloride. The African-American doctor came in with three followers. "We had seen him at Amherst-remember, Mom?"

Her face was swollen and her checks were red like she had been in the sun or under a sun lamp. The pharmacist came in and questioned her; may send her home with a prescription for Dilaudid pain patch. She had calmed down. The best food is here, the shower, nurses on this floor — the best. In MSMH, the food is the worse, the soup is lukewarm water, the canned beans/vegetables are putrid, food tastes frozen, food from can is awful — why? Don't hospitals (like MSMH) realize that people are just laying there sick and look forward to something good during their stay and it's the food?

1:00 p.m.

Debra is being discharged today and that we should take our time coming for her BUT that there was a Farmer's Market in the RPCI park until 2:00 p.m. We were having lunch and couldn't get there by 2:00. At 2:30 p.m. Deb was discharged and sent home with two prescriptions and instructions to keep an eye on how she feels. If she had any unusual pains or any other symptoms, she was given a phone number to call the GYN Clinic until 4:00 p.m. and an emergency number after that time with a 24-hour doctor on staff. (*Really? Amazing!*) We arrived at 3:00 and she was discharged at 3:20 p.m.

Debra, a landscape designer, wanted to stop in the garden, she noticed the beautiful Fountain & Reflection Pond sign and walked toward it. She became excited and laughed as she noticed it was donated by Upstate Pharmacy, "her" pharmacy, she said! "I knew there was a reason to stop and see this. It's so beautiful here!" ⚓ ⚓ However, when we had reached those few steps, I could hear that she was winded and instead of walking with us back through the garden, across the street to the parking lot, I said, "Debra, you sit on the picnic bench with Jerr, and I will go and get the car and pick you guys up."

"Do you want to come home with us, Debra?" "No, Mum, I want to go to Lisa's."

We drove her to Niagara Falls via the NYS Thruway and Grand Island. (*When we passed the exit for Country Glenn, she looked out the window and said, "Boy, I really loved that apartment. Too bad I couldn't keep it after my accident. Maybe I can go back there. Would you guys help me furnish it again?" "Of course, Debra, you had your apartment so neat and cute. Jeremy loved it there with the woods and country walks."*)

As we went from Williams Road to Six Corners, we happened on an major accident between a car and a motorcycle near Tim Horton's. She said, "God bless those people; I know what it feels to have an accident." During the trip home, I noticed that she kept adjusting the seat belt because of the pain in her back. We finally got to Lisa's about 5:00 p.m. and arrived home at 6:30 and both of us fell asleep for an hour. (*When did we ever do that?*)

9/1/11, Thurs., 9:30 p.m. —

Debra feels terrible; she is extremely tired and so weak; she can't even walk; the pain in her back is still there. She got up to eat a bite but didn't want anything else. She can feel the stuff (the chemo fluids) in her body; it's kind of a burning feeling but not pain as such.

L: Are you drinking a lot of water to flush out your bladder as instructed, Deb?

D: Yes, I did remember I have to do that.

L: Let us know how you're doing tomorrow. Lisa has our phone numbers in case she has to call us? If you need us, call any time of the day or night. "I love you two." " *We love you sweetheart.*"

Upstate delivers Omeprazole DR 20 mg

9/2/11, Fri. —

Debra slept most of the day.

Upstate delivers Dexamethasone 4 mg.

9/3/11, Sat. —

Debra is feeling a little better; she gets slightly winded. She has heartburn and takes her Prilosec which was delivered to her immediately after she called. The chemo can give you heartburn; she has back pain; took anti-nausea pills; took them without instruction but felt that's what she should do. She has no joint pain this time. A ditzy pharmacist informed her she can only get the pills for 30 days.

Personal: Jeremy is attending Cheektowaga Central; he is on football team.

"Oh, Mom, I was looking out the window and saw a large mother deer and two does, little ones with white speckles, they were eating the apples on the ground and the mom was picking them off the tree." Debra very quietly and slowly walked back there, but then the mom sensed her and they all took off. When she was walking the short distance to the back yard, she realized she was winded.

"Mummy, there must be a nest in the tree because when a hawk tried to get to it about 50 black birds flew in and were screeching, just like real screams, and then finally the hawk took off. What a wonderful day it was. It reminds me of the times I spent with Jeremy in a park, sitting under a tree and talking for hours and hours. I even have a tiny frame of the park. It reminds me of those times." (*Thank, you, Jesus, for the gift of the most simple and beautiful things in Your world.*)

9/4/11, Sun., 4:45 p.m. @NFMMH —

Debra was taken to the hospital by ambulance. It started during the night, she had pain in her left neck and when she rubbed it, it was wet. When she got up, there was blood all over. The large mole on her neck had blown up, it looked like a sponge, and it was bleeding. She hadn't felt well since that morning. Then about 2:00 p.m. she was sitting on her bed, she started to sweat; she thought that it was the air conditioning unit in her room was not on a high enough setting. Then she was soaking wet, just dripping, it was a cold sweat, she had difficulty breathing and was very weak. She thought "OK, this is affecting my heart again"; then she had a bad pain in her chest and she called 911. No one was home at the time.

Unexpectedly, Colton's friends had come over to pick something up from him, and she said "Don't get scared, there's an ambulance coming for me." They were so concerned, so nice and asked, "What can we do, Debra?"

Debra called us from the E/R; the doctor said she was going to be admitted. The mole that had burst was abscessed; he was calling in a surgeon, and they were going to remove it. The infection was what caused her blood to drop; they are giving her antibiotics.

Personal: In the meantime, Jeremy had called her; he and Phil had been doing a job (carpet install) for Smokin' Joe's (on the Reservation), and they had just finished. He was so excited and proud of his work with his dad. She quietly told Jeremy how wonderful he was and that she would call him back; she didn't tell him she was in the hospital.

Lorr: Did you leave Lisa a note? We want to come to the hospital.

Debra: No, I'll call her cell phone later. Lisa is going to her dentist; she hadn't been going regularly; and when Lisa met my dentist, she loved her. The dentist asked about Debra and that they were waiting for her to come back after her treatments.

Debra said the removal of the mole was on her "To Do" list and could now be crossed off! "See there are angels around me, Mom."

"Debra, I have noticed that another little mole was growing right below the other one."

Debra said, "I know. Now they can take care of both of them at the same time. I always thought it was from my necklace rubbing. "

She had a great breakfast; when the tray came, she expected a yucky one but there were scrambled eggs, toast, fruit, cereal and beverages — bring this chef back!

Her back hurts. She said she must have slept wrong or twisted it somehow or maybe sleeping wrong? Or some other way.

9/5/11, Mon, — Labor Day @NFMMH —

Chris called that Debra wants me to call her hospital room as her cell phone battery is dead, and she didn't remember to take her charger in the urgency of calling 911. She can't call anybody on her hospital phone, as calls to Chris, Lisa, and us are considered long distance; the phone is only for local calls.

She's on the 4th Floor. The EKG was OK. More blood tests were taken; she will be given platelets or blood transfusions and antibiotics. The E/R and the hospital was packed, but she was taken to her room in two hours. She's waiting for her pain meds and awaiting an answer from the doctor. Her nurse gave Debra a back rub, then gave her sandwiches because she hadn't eaten all day. The doctor came in just as she was being given a dinner tray. Debra asked me to call Colton's friend on his cell phone and ask him to go to Lisa's and feed the dogs. It was going on 8:30 p.m. and they were supposed to eat at 6:00. When I called him, he asked 'How's Debra doing?'

She's being given pain shots every six hours, but they stopped them because her blood pressure dropped; they are waiting for doctor, but the nurses are changing shifts, the pain in her back is like a knife and it doesn't go away. She was sobbing when I talked to her. (*I asked her what I can do. Why can't we come to the hospital?*)

D: Nothing, Mom! I'm being taken care of; I don't want you to make the long trip here. I asked for pain meds at 3:00 P.M.

Jerr: *"Let's go anyway, what can she do — throw us out of the room?"*

"Jerr, I've seen Debra get upset when people don't do what she wants; let's respect her wishes for right now." I called the nurses' station and asked when she would get her meds. The nurse said, "The order is being filled right now."

Personal: Chris fell down the stairs on Friday, he was wearing socks and now his back is screwed up. She felt she should have been there for him.

7:30 p.m. —

I talked to Debra and she still hadn't given her pain meds, and she was in so much pain.

At 8:30 p.m. —

There was a different nurse who said the doctor was in E/R. Debra was crying; she was given blood transfusions — two bags so far.

Dr. Kali, the surgeon, came in and explained he would perform the surgery tomorrow, her mole *(about the size of a dime, I guessed)* was a "skin tag" and he would snip it off and will also remove the smaller one below it. The moles will be sent to Pathology. Her blood chemistry is only up a point off 10/7. She asked us to call her later tonight.

10:05 p.m. —

When I called, the operator told me all phones to the patient rooms were shut off for the evening. I asked to speak to the 4th Floor nurses' station. When I finally reached Debra's nurse, Kate, I asked how she was going; she said she was better. "Has she been given her pain meds?" "No, not that I'm aware." I asked why she hadn't been given pain meds; she said I just gave it to her at 8:00 p.m. "I said, 8:00? She's been asking for pain meds since 3:00 and now it's 8:00 - that's five hours!" She said, "I don't know what the other nurse did." *(Well, obviously — nothing.)*

L: *Isn't it in the computer?*

Nurse: She looked and said, yes, she was given pain meds at 4:00; you have to scan it when you take it out of the drawer.

L: *I can't understand why at 7:30, Debra told me she hadn't been given pain meds.*

Nurse: She said she would be comfortable in about one hour.

L: *Since 8:00 p.m. That doesn't sound right. Please help me understand and help my daughter.*

Nurse: I've had a call in for the doctor who was in the building.

(I record everything Debra tells me and everything the doctors are telling her and that she had asked for pain med at 3:00 p.m. I talked to her at 5:00 p.m. and she still didn't have it. Then at 7:00 p.m. and still no meds and now I was trying to get her again and didn't know all the phones were turned off at 10:00.)

Nurse: That's always been the rule.

(We didn't know that. But if you said she was given pain meds at 4:00, then something is strange. I thanked her for the information and to please tell Debra that I had tried to reach her.)

9/6/11, Tues. —

Debra's phone was busy all morning, couldn't get through. Then after lunch there was still no answer. *What happened, did she go home?*

6:30 p.m.

Chris called and said Debra wanted me to call her. The surgery on her neck took two seconds, the preparation took longer. Afterwards, the doctor came in and explained about the pain meds she was being given. They can't give her pain meds by IV; it drops her blood pressure too much. He increased two pain pills more frequently — from six hours to every four hours, OxyContin*; her white blood counts are down.

A female pain management doctor came and talked to Debra about treatment; she said nerve pain is sometimes a side effect of chemo treatments. She was ordering Cymbalta* for nerve pain, but that would affect her mood; also morphine pills. Debra doesn't think she'll be able to continue on that med. when discharged and doesn't want to. (*Thank, God, we were told and had read that pain meds were not addictive in cancer cases.*) Antibiotics every four hours. The nurses said Ifosemide had no side effects! Even the goofy pharmacist said the same thing.

9/7/11, Wed., 10:30 a.m. @ MSMH —

Called Debra before we went to Lewiston. She was in pain in her stomach; it was burning, and she was writhing in pain, and crying, asked if the doctor was still on the floor, she wanted to see her. The doctor ordered a CT scan on her stomach. They are keeping the pain meds to every four hours and it takes the edge off the back pain. Lidocaine patches don't work! She needs pain meds before it gets bad.

9:00 p.m.

Doctor ordered Lyrica 75 mg-Gabatraten. The nurse was questioning the doctor's decision! She was real bitchy. Tried to say that Lortab the same as Dilaudid! (*NOT!*) Debra told us, "Please, Mom, I don't want company and I don't want you and Jerr to see me like this. I'm miserable!" (*Well, I guess it was a good thing because I felt like wiping up the hospital with their pain management methods! We just don't understand these procedures. And pain management signs are posted everywhere! Every hospital it takes forever to get relief!*)

9/8/11, Thurs. - 2:30 p.m. —

Debra's really sick, the nurse was just there; she's getting her meds.

6:30 p.m. —

Debra very sick; waiting for doctor to adjust her meds; they are giving her morphine; she may have shingles again. Everything is fine; she didn't eat dinner; she can't eat anything and was sleeping as much as possible. She doesn't know about the results of CT scan or whether she has shingles again.

She was upset that I called again, doesn't want us there! The hospital won't let us stay anyway. Her words are slurred, and I don't feel she really knows I called. She doesn't know anyone's name. When the nurse told her the Dilaudid and Lortab were the same, she told that same nurse she's not here to argue with her but she asked to speak to the doctor.

"Mom, I can't hold the phone, I'm writhing in pain, I'm miserable. Please don't call the hospital, the nurses, or the doctor. I asked for pain meds two hours ago. I don't have good nurses today; told the nurse it's not up to her to dispense my meds. I need to speak to the doctor again."

(I'm sick; I'm crying; I'm pacing the floor, and all Jerr can do is stop me and hold me. What can I do? Who can I call? Why isn't there a hospital "police" or advocate to whom you can complain. Where do we turn? Then Debra says some nurses find a way to retaliate if we complain.)

9/9/11, Fri., 12:20 p.m. —

Hasn't had her lunch yet; feeling slightly better, she feels like she has a cold, she was shivering during the night, got up to go to bathroom and was cold and she got under a blanket. Then she was sweating and had a fever from the platelets. The doctor said, "I don't really see breakout from shingles; it might be nerve damage from the chemo. CT scan doesn't show anything, but you have an infection somewhere."

Personal: Donna called Debra, she got a speeding ticket, said she was feeling "just peachy keen." *(Really? And I am, Mom?)*

4:30 p.m.

Debra called us! She was all excited! (She had called the hospital operator and asked how she could make calls and the operator told her how and also said she/we may be charged long distance charges.) She's looking out her window and sees the pilots rehearsing for the Niagara Air Show this weekend, they are flying low, turning loops, going sideways and sometimes, becoming almost invisible. She told Chris the same thing that she has a bird's eye view of the Air Show. "What a gift, Mom, and people form lines for hours and then try to find parking, and then a spot to sit. And here I have an unobstructed view, a front row seat! You could be up there, Mom." *Oh, sure, with the Blue Angels?!* 🛫 🛫

7:30 p.m. —

Debra's feeling much better; they started giving her the medicine for shingles yesterday but only after Dr. Shank, the pain management doctor, stormed out of her room to speak to the nurses! Debra was crying and writhing in pain, didn't even eat her meals. Today, the doctor peeked around the door and said, "Are you speaking to me, Debra? They did not want to hear from me yesterday (nurses/doctors?). Your smile just made my day."

Debra: The pain was so sharp and stabbing, you just want to reach and rip out the part that hurts.

Dr. Shank: I know how you feel, Debra. I suffered with Fibromyalgia, and no one would believe me until it was finally diagnosed. So I **do** know what you are talking about.

Debra told the doctor that the nurses aren't listening to her and that she knows what she's talking about. After all this time, she knows her own body and what is the cause of her pain. She's had to self-diagnose herself these past two years. She hates the morphine; it makes her vomit, and it doesn't help the pain. She had different nurses today and they didn't treat her any differently because of the situation yesterday. She's sure the "word" was passed. *(What a pity that patients are at the mercy of a medical professional's bias or moods or anything that bothers them and if we say anything, there is payback for the patient.)*

9/10/11, Sat. —

Debra is feeling much better. We called first and then stopped
to visit her on our way back from the Kiwanis Peach Festival in
Lewiston. We brought her huge peach shortcake without the
whipped cream. ⬆️ ⬆️ But we stopped at the grocery store and
bought a can of Extra Creamy Whipped Cream, and her shortcake
was loaded with cold whipped cream a foot high when we walked
in! The smile on her face brought out the sunshine for us. We left
the can because the shortcake was so big, she would need a second
or third squirt! When we finally left, she was saying, "Yummy."
Later, she used it for her midnight snack!

Dr. Hanaan came in while we were there. She is a wonderful
person. Dr. Hanaan told us she has 236 days left and then will hang
out a shingle for Family Practice. She is staying in the area because
she has a beautiful house which doesn't cost her very much; it has
beautiful mahogany floors. When she told us the address, I knew it
was one of the old, historic homes in Niagara Falls.

Debra said the nurse was again arguing or questioning the doctor
when she wanted to give Debra Dilaudid and kept questioning
the meds.

Debra's sodium chloride beeper went off and the nurse didn't
answer. Then Deb's heart monitor became unplugged; and again,
the nurse didn't answer. No one answered at 3:30 p.m. when Debra
asked for a pain shot, she called her a few times. Betts, an aide
came instead and said, "The nurse was very busy doing patient
reports, you know." Deb finally got her pain shot at 4:30 p.m. and
shortly after, she seemed to nod off and we left. (*I was seething;
'reports' is more important than 'patients'? When did nurses become so
computer-oriented that patient care was second in importance, I thought.
Jerr says they have such long hours, so much to do, so many patients. Well,
Jerr, it's only my daughter I'm worried about.*)

9:50 p.m. —

Debra was finally comfortable! When it was time for another shot, her evening nurse, Ken, was right there with it. He brought her a snack and ginger ale. She needs to have sodium chloride before pain meds. "Mom, what a gift Ken is. I never have to ask for anything, he's right there on time with my doses and anything else I want." (*Thank you, God.*)

9/11/11, Sun. —

I went to the 9/11 Memorial Ceremony at Williamsville Town Hall. When I got home, there was a message from Debra not to come to the hospital until she called again.

3:00 p.m. —

I called Debra at 3:00 p.m. She's being discharged. Chris is coming to pick her up, she needs to go to his house to get some paperwork for Social Security. Her boxes are stored in his attic, and it needs to be done ASAP. If Social Security calls, they need to know how sick she's been, that she has nerve pain in her hands and feet and that sometimes can't feel whether she's holding a cup or glass of liquid or doesn't feel her sneakers on her feet. The nurse called for transportation, but that it would take one hour. Chris cannot wait so says he hopes she will be ready in one hour; he was having a band practice at the house.

"Debra, can we come to pick you up? We're happy to do so."

"Mom, I don't want you guys to drive one hour to get me, when Chris is five minutes away. I don't want you to do that. We'll talk later."

9/12/11, Mon., 6:00 p.m. — Debra's call

When I returned her call at 8:00 p.m., we talked until 9:00.

Personal: "Chris picked me up from the hospital; I found the records I needed in his attic, and Lisa came to pick me up. Chris has been buying so many items for the house — why?"

Personal: For Jeremy's birthday, he wants the earring. She has a stone she can have reset and take him to the Mall to have it done. "Will you take us, Mom? I need to do this for him. I promised him when he was 13 that he could have one when he turned 16. Then maybe can we go to Lasertron. Chris wants to come and will pay his own way. I will call Lasertron and find out the cost of admission."

9/19/11, Mon. —

Chris drove Debra to us for her next chemo at RPCI tomorrow. Her pain management doctor told her she has nerve damage from the chemo; it is called postherpetic neuralgia*. Her appointment with the doctor is on 12/7/11 and she doesn't want to miss it. Dr. Kanaan is going to ask Dr. LaiLai for a prescription for Lyrica 75 mg which Debra has taken before.

Personal: We talked about Chris; about Mark going through chemotherapy and Sally's condition with her failing eyesight. Debra said, "Mom, Mark better be sensitive as to how he feels and needs to call 911 if he gets to the point that I did. If you want me to talk to him, Mom, I will. Have him read all the material they give him if they give him the books, pamphlets, etc."

8:30 p.m. — @ E/R MFSH

Debra became ill with chest pain and pain in her muscles. It became progressively worse, and we finally took her in. X-rays were taken and blood work done. She was finally discharged at 1:30 a.m. with the usual medication instructions to continue hydroquinone-acetaminophen (Lortab 10/500 every 6 hours as needed. She was also given a print-out explanation of Chest Wall Pain and a diagnosis as Pleuritic chest pain; Musculoskeletal chest pain.

2:30 a.m. — I heard Debra sobbing in her bedroom. I went in and she told me, "I can't do this anymore, Mummy, I can't do this anymore, I just can't do this anymore. The only thing that keeps me going is Jeremy. I want to see him graduate, I want to see him enter the Police Academy, I want to see him find a nice girl and get married and have a good life. But I just can't do this any more." We cried together, I held her and rocked her in my arms. I stayed with her stroking her face and her soft, fuzzy hair until she fell asleep. I then put my hands over her and prayed, "Please, God, let this be true — somehow, that she gets to see her goals for her son, Jeremy. But in all things, Thy will be done. Be merciful, oh, Lord. "

9/20/11, Tues. — @ RPCI 8:00 a.m. appt.

Chemo treatment: Ifosfamide

Debra's second admission for the three-day Ifosfamide treatment.

At 7:00 a.m. (*I never went back to bed after comforting Debra*), I quietly woke Jerr, and he readied his meds, shots, etc. and I prepared him a small breakfast. At 8:15 a.m., I woke Debra, she had her toast breakfast, and we left for Buffalo. In spite of what her schedule stated, Dr. LaiLai didn't remember she was being admitted, so another doctor examined Debra.

Because of the room overflow, Debra was put on 6th Floor North-PEDIATRICS! There was only a small boy and a teenager in that section with three nurses. Now she was laughing and said, "Mom, it figures that I'd end up here!" She was delighted with the color-ful pictures, the butterflies hanging from the ceilings, the happy symbols on all the doors instead of numbers. She loved the door to her room with a huge smiling sun face on it, and especially the Parents Room. She immediately began to make plans to have Jeremy visit her, and they would have dinner together and make popcorn in the kitchen, then curl up together and watch videos in the Parents Room.

9/22/11

Upstate delivers Lyrica 75 mg.

Date	DAY/TIME	LOCATION	SCHEDULED PROCEDURE	NOTES	COMPLETED	NURSE
9/20/11	Tues.	RPCI- Buffalo	Phlebotomy Unit	Ifosfamide, chemo	Yes	Debbie
	9:00 a.m.	6th Floor North Pediatrics!	Check-in	Daladid		Lucia-secr.
	9:30 a.m.		CGYN-(Dr. LaiLai)	Lortabs		
	9:45 a.m.		Room #617	Cheeks swollen and bright red		
	10:45 a.m.			Slight arms palsy		
				Talkative after med.		
				Food yummy		
				Nights very quiet, Lovely finally!		
				Nurses right on target with pain meds. every 4 hours		

Date	DAY/TIME	LOCATION	SCHEDULED PROCEDURE	NOTES	COMPLETED	NURSE
9/21/11	Wed.		Visit from Pain Mgmt. Team	Lyrica 75 mg for nerve pain		Lisa ☺
				Cheeks swollen and bright red		Sarah 🔼
				Slight arms palsy		Lucia
				Talkative after med		
				Food yummy		
				Told us about the Farmers Market in the garden		

9/22/11, Thurs. — @ RPCI —

I spoke to Phil about Jeremy's birthday, and he agreed with Jeremy getting his ears pierced and the earring. Debra then had a candid conversation with Phil about her treatment and repeated the story that Jeremy was the reason she kept going. She was sobbing. He was very empathetic, and while Debra sobbed, they told each other that each of them were the reason Jeremy was such a great kid, good in school, knows what he wants to do, doesn't cause trouble, very mature. Phil may bring Jeremy to our house on Friday and may come to his birthday event at Lasertron on Saturday.

Debra wants to try a stop at the wig center; hopefully, we can get something instead of her black wig (*Her girlfriend, a photography student, gave her the black wig when she asked Debra to model for her black and white photo shoot.*)

In the morning, she had a hilarious conversation with Lisa about where she was and the food she could order! 🔼 🔼

When a crowd of doctors came into her room, she asked the

pain doctor about the difference between him and a neurologist? He said there isn't any difference. One female Indian doctor was very abrupt and talked over her answers; she didn't really listen to Debra, then she stated there was no way Debra could have shingles without the blisters outside and that a CT scan wouldn't show shingles! Another doctor quietly told Debra, "Yes, you can have shingles without breaking out in blisters externally." Debra said, "I know. A doctor in the Niagara Falls found it. They did find it, and I didn't have the outbreak of external blisters. They found all the blisters inside through a CT scan and prescribed Lyrica 75 mg for me. Please, I don't want to leave the hospital without a prescription for Lyrica 75 mg." The one doctor said she would have it. *"Does anyone stop to realize that kindness is like a pebble tossed in a lake and the ripples go on forever?! The same is true, Debra, of hurtful words and actions!"*

Personal: :Mom, I want to take Jeremy to the Boulevard Mall to get his earrings. Everybody — Phil and Chris — and whoever showed up would pay for their own admission."

9/23/11, Fri. — @ RPCI —

Debra was discharged around 3:30 p.m. and all of us walked to the Buffalo Medical Group building to pick up Mark, having his own chemo treatment, dropped him off at his home in Kenmore and then came home. Debra said she wanted to go home that night because all her clothes and wig were there; she hadn't brought them with her. So I drove her to North Tonawanda to meet up with Lisa.

9/24/11, Sat. - 11:00 a.m.

Debra told us that Phil had wanted to drop Jeremy off at 1:30 p.m. She was resting; originally he had said 6:00 p.m., but OK. We ended up picking her up at 4:30 p.m., and Phil and Jeremy finally dropped over at 6:30 p.m. as we were getting dinner ready. We had a quick but nice visit for thirty minutes, invited Phil to stay for dinner,

but he kept looking at his watch, saying, "I've got to get home."
We had a wonderful dinner with Debra and Jeremy, who stayed
overnight with us. What a pleasure!

9/26/11, Mon., 11:00 a.m. —

A momentous day, Jeremy's sixteenth birthday! Then Debra,
Jeremy and I drove to the Boulevard Mall to get Jeremy's ears
pierced and earring at Claire's, however, a glitch! According to NYS
laws, because he was underage, Debra's permission was needed
and they asked to see her ID. She didn't have her wallet so I drove
back to Williamsville to pick it up.

12:00 —

I arrived back at the Boulevard Mall and at last, Jeremy finally got
his ears pierced. I was panicking and nervous and walked out of
the store. Jeremy was embarrassed with my nervousness. I was
pretending to cover my eyes, peeking through my fingers outside
the window. (*Remember, I'm a chicken and have a dread of needles. Do
you know how big those needles are? Well, they are with your eyes closed!*
⚓ *Then I bought Debra a wallet she could carry! We laughed because it
was a Hello Kitty one.*) I paid for the piercing and earrings and we
drove to Lasertron. No one showed up and after waiting for a time,
we finally went in and registered.

1:00 p.m. —

Found out the Lasertron experience would be three hours, about
one hour for each game. Jeremy signed up for a Lasertron tag
inside and the racing carts outside.

1:15 p.m. Laser Tag — Briefing time

2:00 p.m. Bought pizza and drinks in between the 15 minute break
they gave us.

2:12 p.m. Go Kart (2 races)

2:52 p.m. Go Kart (2 races)

3:30 p.m. Finished about 3:30 p.m. and got home at 4:00.

Outside on the racetrack, Jeremy and Debra kept racing around and around in their cars, Debra in her cap and her wig flying around her shoulders, and Jeremy looking back to see her catching up with him. Big grins and lots of laughter. I kept watching Debra to see how she was coping, but she was glowing. She had a happy face and a grin about everything, especially about the delight Jeremy was having experiencing something his Mom had promised him. "Thank you for everything, Mom. You have made us so happy today. We love you two." "Grandma, thank you for everything, love ya."

As we were preparing for dinner, Lisa called unexpectedly that she was at Wal-Mart in Amherst with her mother and could we take Debra and Jeremy there, so she could drive them back earlier than planned. She didn't want to make a second trip. So here I go back to Niagara Falls Blvd. and dropped them off with Lisa. Lots of hugs and kisses. Jerr and I returned home, fell asleep and missed the 5:00 pills and the start of 6:00 dinner! *("Us'ns are getting too old for all this, Pa!" Jerr and I were laughing.)* ⚓ ⚓

10:00 p.m. — Debra's call

Personal: "Phil had so explanation as to why the "no show" for Jeremy's Lasertron gift. Also, that Kurt won't let me take my car from his outside parking lot because I don't have enough money to pay him for renting the "air" to store my car!" We paid for it.

9/28/11

Upstate delivers Omeprazole DR 20 mg

10/4/11, Tues., 11:00 a.m. @ E/R NFMMH

Debra is having difficulty breathing, very difficult; she asked Lisa to call 911. A sonogram was just performed and blood tests taken. An ultrasound will be done to determine if she has a blood clot. Debra thinks maybe because of all the stress with everyone's situation affected her. *"Yes!"* Lisa heard the doctor say Debra cannot be under any stress.

She also received her RPCI appointment sheet for the blood test and exam includes admission again into Pediatrics. *(I asked at the RPCI Hospitality Desk for the telephone number for Patient Advocate; was given the name of Adrien or Carol. Debra has not been given the records she has requested. I left message, never got a call back. Why?)*

10/5/11, Wed. — @ NFMMH

Debra was admitted at 11:30 p.m. after 12 hours in the E/R. She is being given platelets and blood transfusions; her chemistry this time was registered at 5! The doctor is so annoying, just stares at her as if she doesn't know what she's saying, Dr. Newbaum or something, he doesn't listen to her. They gave her the wrong dosage of Lyrica, only gave her one pill a day instead of three pills, and she now has the pain in her back again.

Lisa called Charron and asked if Debra could be brought to RPCI and Charron said, "No, we don't have an emergency room." We wondered why she couldn't be admitted for the blood transfusion.

Later, I asked Dr. LaiLai why RPCI didn't have an emergency room since Debra's symptoms were all cancer related and the doctors there would know how to treat her. All the doctors in other hospitals were guessing and trialing treatments until they were able to reach his office. He answered, "Because then we would have to let anybody in from the neighborhood just for colds or any minor complaints."

(My thought was RPCI patients are given the green embossed plastic cards, and they have to be shown every time they enter RPCI. Could these green cards not be used for emergency treatments? And RPCI is right next

*door to Buffalo General, and we understand there's even a tunnel between
the two hospitals! We had the feeling he just didn't want to hear about or
deal with Debra's symptoms.)*

10/6/11, Thurs. —

Debra is feeling very tired, the blood cultures still aren't ready;
the doctor said there's an infection somewhere, maybe in the port
which may have to be removed and reinserted! The doctor was
so mad because he said somebody hadn't done their job properly.
Debra feels like she has a cold or the flu, when did she get her last
flu shot? Her joints, shoulders, and knees hurt. She is still being
given antibiotics, sodium chloride, blood transfusion and pain
shots. Her nurse is wonderful. Later in the evening, a male nurse
was so caring to her and he remembered her from RPCI and asked
her, "What are you doing here, Debbie?" Her fever is 101°.

She had the most delicious grilled fish, thinks it was haddock,
zucchini, baked potato, lemon meringue pie. I asked her whether
she was telling people that the Social Security representative said
she was in Stage 4? Debra hesitated for a minute, then said, "Yes,
Mommy, that's what they told me, but it's not the same Stage 4
as other cancers, it only means that in my case, it's the method of
treatment I am receiving." *I accepted that — why?*

10/7/11, Fri. — @ NFMMH

Dr. Lee came in and asked how she was feeling. Her blood cultures
are not ready. She is on antibiotics. Debra called RPCI (Charron)
who said to let her know how she is doing as she was concerned.
Charron gave Debra the name and phone number of Patient
Advocate at RPCI because Social Security still hasn't received
her medical reports! Charron stated, "You probably won't reach
anybody until Tuesday, when you are scheduled to be admitted
anyway." Debra has already signed a release. At NFMMH, she was
informed that they wouldn't bring her records up to her room but

said when she was discharged, she could stop at the 1st floor and ask for them. (*We did and never got them.*)

10/8/11, Sat. — @ NFMMH

Jerr and I drove to Niagara Falls to see Debra. Nothing new, still being given all the same meds., Dr. Lee said again blood cultures still not ready. We left there before dark, crossing the street and into the creepy parking ramp.

10/9/11, Sun. — @ NFMMH

Debra, "Mommy, I'm glad you woke me up, my legs were crossed, and now I can't feel them or get out of bed! I need to move." She is still being given antibiotics; the nurse had her spit in a cup yesterday, chest pain is not as bad. "Mom, would I have a virus? It still hurts by my breast bone." The doctor has been in to see her yet.

Personal: She laughed, "It's a good day for Jeremy and Colton to go hunting, they are so serious and careful with their rifles and only use areas that properly belong to either Doug or Phil. Jeremy has taken shot gun hunting classes, and they have to go with an adult."

Dr. Lee finally came in and told her he has identified what she has and it's pneumonia! He's glad they have been giving her antibiotics, and Deb was glad they didn't send her home without knowing what was wrong. She had a pneumonia shot last year, and it's supposed to be good for 10 years, so what gives? She remembers again when Jeremy had pneumonia and we didn't know it.

"Debra, it (the pneumonia) came in charging on the white horse you always wanted and attacked you, lady!" We were laughing and she said, "Finally, doctors know what is wrong and can treat it. Yeeeah!" 🛳️ 🛳️

8:30 p.m. — @ NFMMH

Dinner was a cold cut sub, however, she removed the chicken because it was slimy; she only ate the roast beef. Whatever they are giving her is making her go to the bathroom with very little notice, sometimes almost doesn't make it. She asked if she could be transferred by ambulance to RPCI if she's not discharged by Tuesday. "Mom, I have to make that appointment. I will also see how if it would be more convenient for me to get to Buffalo — either Lisa from Niagara Falls or you. I will have to let you know."

"It doesn't matter, sweetheart, we'll manage. We love you." "I love you two, too."

10/10/11, Mon. — @ NFMMH

Another day in the hospital. Dr. Lee said she he is giving her a different antibiotic for the pneumonia; she is so tired; blood culture, sweating a lot (*Good, I think. Doesn't that mean the pneumonia is breaking up?*). Her nurse Dawn told Debra she will call RPCI (Charron) and tell her Debra's still in the hospital. Charron returned the call to Debra that her admission has been changed to Thursday She is to go to the Amherst Clinic first at 10:30 a.m. where a chest x-ray will be done on the 1st floor, then blood work on 2nd, then an internal exam by Dr. LaiLai who will determine if she's well enough to be admitted to RPCI that same day. Also that to administer chemo while she still has pneumonia will put her "at risk". She had a turkey sandwich, her favorite, from the Grateful Deli for lunch.

10/11/11, Tues. — Scheduled Chemo treatment cancelled.

10/11/11, Tues., 5:00 p.m. — @ NFMMH

Debra is spitting phlegm but it's clear white, not yellow or green. She is being given a different kind of antibiotic; she's very, very tired.

Debra is watching the construction outside her window in front of hospital and said: "Mom, if I were an inspector, this crew would get numerous violations for safety hazards, careless work, etc. and the workers are so slow and lazy, and apparently no one is overseeing the work. And, Mom the same little street has been worked on since a year ago when I was here! (*I know, the entrance to the crummy parking garage is blocked and there are potholes, really poor impression of Niagara Falls' only hospital. In the garage, there's a crudely handwritten sign taped to the wall with masking tape to stop at the booth to pay fee, but there has never been anyone in the booth. We looked all over for a place to pay the parking fee and there was nothing. Then the lanes direct you to exit at the rear of the garage where there's a locked gate and no way of raising the arm. So you back up into another lane and try to leave at the entrance you came in. A real mess.*) We agree with Debra, "They have been doing this for over a year while we've been coming here. There doesn't appear to be any progress, broken concrete all over the street, no proper sidewalks, no caution signs."

For meals, Debra usually orders cold sandwiches because the food is inedible; she looked forward to the bowl of 'fruit in season' she ordered and got canned fruit cocktail!

"Mummy, please look up when the Apple Festival is in Lockport. I want to take Jeremy there; it's one of our favorites." *Honey, you don't want to do to Pumkinfest in Clarence but come to our house first? "* Oh, gosh, no, Mom, because this is closer to home if I get sick."

10/12/11, Wed. @ NFMMH

Debra: "Nothing new; I'm still here. My doctor told me they were still checking my bacteria levels. My nurse is Karren. When I called RPCI , Charron wasn't in the Office today, but I was referred to Tammy or Kris, however, as usual had to leave a message on the voice mail to call me." (**Never received a call back.**)

7:20 p.m. — Debra's call

One doctor told her she would still be there tomorrow and the other doctor said she was going to be transferred to RPCI tomorrow. (*How?*) So she said, "I'll see what they do with me, Mom, but don't come to the hospital today until I find out." She has the pain in her back; she's going to ask to see a nerve doctor; it is in such an different, awkward spot that she can't reach and sometimes it helps to have pressure put on it with a rolled up pillow or something, but she can't keep it there long. Even with the Lyrica 75 mg, it doesn't help the pain now. The doctor said her blood chemistries are good enough but that RPCI has different standards.

Personal: Lisa still has her cough, thinks she has bronchitis and is getting an antibiotic.

10/13/11, Thurs., a.m. @ NFMMH

The doctor doesn't know if she's going to RPCI today; she still has her fever; she fell asleep and woke up breaking out in sweat. Debra still feels like she has the flu.

P.M. — No change, still waiting to see what they are going to do. The doctor came and said he doesn't know what's happening either. Is she going to RPCI next week? They don't do chemo on weekends so there's no use her being transferred there tomorrow! Why don't they tell her?

Personal: Debra called that Donna was having car problems again, everybody was involved.

10/14/11, Fri. — @ NFMMH

"Mom, today is Chris' birthday and I can't call him. My phone is out of battery, and I forgot to take the cord again. How sad I am not to be there to surprise him and bake one of my special cakes. Please ask him try to reach me through the hospital phone."

10/15/11, Sat. —

Debra was discharged but still feels wobbly and has been sleeping. Chris came to pick her up. I talked to Chris, and he said that nothing special happened for his birthday. Laughing, Debra said: "Oh, so you missed my special surprises and silly gifts and birthday cake with funny decorations, huh?" 🎂🎂 He said he didn't know Debra was in the hospital again and wondered why she hadn't called him, so apparently Lisa didn't let him know either.

If she is finally admitted to RPCI, it would be with the arrangements she made to have Jeremy there and they could watch videos.

In the meantime, Debra was nauseated, throwing up every day, shaking, bumping into walls, she was so wired up by all the stress around her. Lisa asked her, "Debra what's wrong with you; you look terrible; you don't want to eat; do you want me to take you back to the hospital?" Debra told her that maybe later but she wanted to try to sleep first.

10/17/11, Mon. —

Debra's appointment at RPCI and after three hours, we finally did go to Perkins Restaurant and of course, Debra ordered her favorite dinner — turkey club.

DATE	DAY/ TIME	LOCATION	SCHEDULED PROCEDURE	NOTES	COMPLETED	NURSE
10/18/11	Tues. 10:00 a.m	Amherst Clinic per Charron Waited 1 hour and were told she was supposed to be at Buffalo.	Radiology Dept.- 1st Floor Phlebotomy Lab Chest x-ray 2nd Floor — Dr. LaiLai Admission to 6 North Pediatrics, Room 6717	Ifosfamide, chemo Dalaudid Lortab Lyrica 75 mg Cheeks swollen and bright red Talkative after med. Food is yummy Nights very quiet — at last. Nurses right on target with pain meds. every 4 hours		Jennifer Lucia-secr.

10/19/11	Wed.	RPCI- Buffalo	*We only visited for one hour because we had Mark at Buffalo General and he needed to be picked up.*	*She's very sleepy; hardly talked to us.* *Later, found out she was sitting on a chair and she fell on floor.* *Did not realize it; all she knew was all of a sudden she was looking up at the bottom of bed and heard the nurse ask if she was alright. She hit her knee pretty hard and slight cut on her leg.*		Lisa ♀ Sarah ☝ Lucia
10/20/11	Thurs.	RPCI- Buffalo	*We drove to Cheektowaga and picked Jeremy up from school and took him to the hospital.*			
10/21/11	Fri.	RPCI- Buffalo	*Talked to Debra at 2:30 and she was in IMCU!*			
10/22/11	Sat.	RPCI- Buffalo	*10:00 a.m.*			Dave
10/23/11	Sun.	RPCI- Buffalo				Sue
10/24/11	Mon.	RPCI- Buffalo				Sue
10/25/11	Tues.	RPCI- Buffalo	*Discharged?*			

10/18/11, Tues. @ RPCI —

Jerr and I stopped at Perkins for dinner after visiting Debra. We were quiet and then at the same moment, we both said, "Debra w......." We missed her not being with us to order her favorite foods.

10/24/11, Mon. @ RPCI —

This was the day that Jeremy was scheduled to visit with Debra in the Pediatrics wing, watch a video in either her room or the Parents Room, and maybe make popcorn in the kitchen. Jerr and I will leave them together and wander around the hospital. We picked Jeremy up from school. At RPCI, a place he had always heard of but had never been to, we showed him the Lobby, then the gift shop where he bought Debra a card and little stuffed animal — guess what? A 'Hello Kitty!' and some "snackies" for himself. (Debra said, "Jeremy always laughed at and loved the word "snackies" ever since our visit to Florida and you said we're having "snackies" for lunch. Jerr asked, "What the heck are 'snackies' and you said it was a word you made up for a light lunch bites because we were going out for dinner!" Lots of laughter over that word.) ⬆⬆ We showed him the 1st floor, the 2nd floor, and then went to the 6th floor, Pediatrics.

When we walked into Debra's room, she had her cap off, was curled in a fetal position and wouldn't open her eyes, and when she did, they rolled back! Nor was she able to talk, she was attempting but words were coming out in mumbles. Later, she told us she saw Jeremy and thought she was talking to him, but she wasn't. I immediately turned around and was on my way to the nurse's station when she hurriedly came walking in. I asked the nurse what happened?! She urged me out in the hallway and quietly said, "Debra was given quite a jolt of chemo and had a reaction from it." She was having what appeared to be seizures and was flailing her arms around. Jeremy picked up a book from the table explaining

"Patient Rights at RPCI" and was pretending to read it. I told Jeremy, the information in that book doesn't apply to your mother because it's all about surgery and the before and after treatment.

I stood by the window looking out, I was shaking. Then through the reflection in the glass, I saw Jeremy's ears getting red and heard him sniffle, and all of a sudden he covered his face and was sobbing. Debra tried to reach for him, but she couldn't. I was crying and so did Jerr have tears. We were all hugging. I talked to Jenn, the nurse, who said, "We've given her meds to bring her out of it, it will take about 30-40 minutes."

We sat around for a few minutes, and then Deb started mumbling, "I feel funny, I feel funny, I have a pain in my stomach, it hurts, and I have a pain." I called the nurse and she came running, took her vitals, and then called the doctor. A doctor arrived within a few minutes (it was not Dr. LaiLai) and examined Debra. He was asking her questions and she wasn't answering. He ordered pain meds for the pain in her stomach. Jenn said sometimes another side affect of the meds is a gas pain, but it's not the kind that can be alleviated by burping or passing gas. She said give us a few minutes with Debra; why don't you take Jeremy for a walk or downstairs to the cafeteria, have dinner and then come back; she'll be OK in a while, give her an hour. The doctor said her electrolytes* were way down and that's what caused the above symptoms.

I told Jeremy what the nurse had told me and reminded him that his mother had been in hospitals many times and when she came out, wasn't she smiling and talking to him and doing special things with him, and that's what's going to happen this time. (Dear, God, please make this so, not only for my beautiful daughter but for her wonderful son.)

We took Jeremy to the cafeteria for dinner, and he and Jerry had quite a conversation about Cuba because Jeremy told us about his Criminal Justice class that day, and that the class was shown a video about minorities — the Mexicans crossing the border and hopping on trains to get across the border. Jerr and I told him a lot about our trips as missionaries to Cuba, about communism and Castro and how Jerr, his mother and two brothers, had come to the United States 55 years ago. It had taken eleven years to have their application approved and then they only had one week's notice and the family could only bring a small suitcase with them.

On the TV in the cafeteria, there was extensive coverage about Khadafy being killed. Jeremy was interested in all the reports and then he asked more questions. He seemed to feel a lot better by the time we finished dinner. When we came out of the cafeteria, there was a pianist playing the grand piano in the Lobby, and we stood on the mezzanine and listened for a while. What a beautiful, calming gift.

When we cautiously walked back into Debra's room, she had a big smile and reached out to Jeremy, "Hi, Pookie, come here, I'm alright." He looked at us, puzzled, but his face just glowed, and he sat by the bed and got her hand and she started talking. Debra told us, "OMG, I felt like I was having a seizure, or like what I imagine a seizure is like, like my head and eyes were rolled back, were they? I knew what I wanted to say but couldn't say anything; it was coming out garbled like my tongue was swollen. When the doctor was asking me questions, in my head, I knew the answers to his questions as to what day is this, what year is it, do I know where I am, etc. But everything was coming out garbled. I could hear what everyone was saying but couldn't respond. Oh, Mom, it was so awful."

Then she realized she didn't have her cap on and thought that must have been a shock for Jeremy because he's never seen her without her cap — not ever in two years. So she calmly asked for her cap, that her head was cold, and I handed to her. It was a NY Yankees cap. Jeremy said, "Yankees? Where did you get that cap?" Debra shrugged her shoulders, and we all laughed. ⚓ ⚓

We talked to Debra for a while; then her dinner came in and it was spaghetti with meat sauce and mashed potatoes, and she said "Oh, yummy." She couldn't sit up to eat. I tried to help feed her but she shook her head and just left it there. She hadn't had lunch either. Then she said she needed to go to the bathroom; she asked me to call the nurse immediately for help. Jenn told Debra she had a foley catheter* and couldn't get out of bed because she hasn't been able to walk, "It's OK, Debbie, you have a foley." She said, "I do? You took it out." Jenne told her, "No, it's still there."

Jerr and I left the room and went back to the gift shop to get Debra some chap stick because her lips were all dry and cracked. Jeremy stayed with her. When we came back in about 20 minutes, Jeremy was leaning down to her; they were talking to each other, holding hands. Dr. LaiLai had just been there and said "No more, Debra, no more will you have this chemo. Never again." He met Jeremy, of course, and later Jeremy was imitating Dr. LaiLai's Indian accent, "No more, Debra, no more will you have this chemo. Never again." We were all laughing, not at what was said but at Jeremy attempting the accent. ⚓

The plan was that Phil was going to pick Jeremy up at the hospital, and we would have left him with his mother to continue their visit, but as were leaving, Phil called Jeremy and said he was working late. So we said, "We'll take you home, sweetheart, whenever you are ready, no rush." We visited with Debra for another hour and then left. When I kissed her goodbye, she whispered, "I'm so glad he (Jeremy) saw me like this, Mummy, the bad and the good. I wouldn't have wanted it, but it happened."

"We love you, sweetheart." Debra: *"I love you both."* When she told Jeremy, "I love you; I'm sorry about our plans being changed." He told her, "I love you, Mom. It's OK." He didn't want to let go of her hand.

I'm shaking, trying to drive home. Highway Route 33 was very dark at night. Jeremy was sitting in the front seat. I told him, "Did you see how fast the doctor came when Jenn called him? Do you think that would have happened in another hospital?" He said, "No." "She's getting good care, Jeremy. Let's just believe in that." When we arrived at his house, Jeremy reached for me, and as I hugged him, I said "You know, Jeremy, it's not a shame to cry, because when you love somebody so much, it comes from the heart. And those tears are a measure of all that love, not a loss of trying to be macho." He hugged me harder, said "I love you" and then he reached to the back to shake Jerr's hand.

Earlier that afternoon, when we had picked Jeremy up at school, it was cold, and he wasn't wearing a jacket, just a tight short sleeve cotton shirt. We realized he had left his sweatshirt at our house, so Jerr gave him his jacket which we had in the trunk. I told him, "It's also not macho not to wear a jacket and then you end up catching a cold." Later, Jerr and I said, "He only has one jacket? Let's go get him one." "You know how kids are, Jerr, he probably has one, he just didn't think to wear it this morning when he left for school (although it was cold already!).

Later that evening when we spoke on the telephone, Debra said, "I was so tired and after I had slept, one of the aides came in and sat and watched TV with me for hours; it was one of those spooky movies. I know you don't like them! What a gift that was, Mummy. And my Jeremy called!" 🛒 🛒

10/24/11, Mon. — @ IMCU RPCI —

My call to the IMCU nurse's station: "I've been trying to get in touch with my daughter and is there a reason she isn't answering her phone?" She asked me to wait just a minute. Then I heard her tell Deb that they are not giving her the Dilaudid by IV; they are giving her Lortab pills, did she want to try a seminal pack? (*No!*) Deb later told me "Sue's the one who tried to tell the pain management interns to change her pain meds last time and now she's doing it again." The interns from pain management were there earlier, and Deb said, "I guess they'd rather give me five pills instead of one IV of Dilaudid." Supposedly the nurse said, "If you are going home, we have to try to wean you off the IV — and because of her "mental state." (*What mental state?!*) They gave her the Dilaudid by IV until 6:30 a.m. She's not being discharged today; she's there for another day. Debra sounds sleepy and not quite with it today, but she said she's OK. We told her we'd be there tomorrow early and will stay for the day.

7:30 a.m. —

Debra called and the doctor hadn't been in yet. We talked again about Jeremy and what had happened and she repeated how she had felt. It does not appear she is going to be discharged on Saturday; she still hasn't been able to walk and when she tried to use the walker, she got dizzy and almost fell. I told her if she was discharged, she could come to us in Williamsville since everybody else (Lisa and company were going to the cabin and taking Jeremy). And that's when she told me that trip wasn't happening. So we'll play it by ear and see what happens.

10:00 a.m. —

She's just getting tubing for blood transfusions, her red blood cells (hemoglobin) are down. Doctor has not been in yet so probably she won't be coming home today.

Debra ate her hard-boiled eggs which were much better than the scrambled eggs; she had sausage, toast, mandarin oranges, and milk. Her legs are not twitching as much, but she hasn't gotten up and walked yet.

She just finished watching a classic movie with Spencer Tracy portraying Thomas Edison when he invented the light bulb. Edison stated he would light up every room from here to Pittsburgh. They offered him $100,000, now he would have gotten over $1 million.

10:30 a.m. — @ RPCI

I called Debra and told her about my research on electrolytes*.
She told me that Dr. LaiLai had just been in, "You're doing good,
Debra, your heart beat is back to normal. Maybe we'll think about
sending you home on Monday."

Personal: Debra told Jeremy about Juliana on eEntertainment, a
beautiful blond; Jeremy knows of her. Debra told me, "She's kind
of flat-chested and she's married to another TV personality. She
and her husband have been trying to get pregnant. Well, she had a
double lumpectomy, has cancer and has been in remission."

4:30 p.m. — @ RPCI

Debra has been going in and out of sleep, but was awake now.
They just started another bag of blood; she's been given Benedryl,
Tylenol, Lyrica 75 mg, and the pain med — Dilaudid. "I'm OK,
Mummy, I'm being taken care of." *"But you don't have Mummy's care,
sweetheart."* "That's true!" 🛁 🛁

"Guess what, Mummy. I ate lunch! All my favorite foods — egg
salad, potato salad, celery sticks, carrots, a plate of real fruit and
peaches." For dinner she ordered roast beef, mashed potatoes, and
green beans. She's already ordered tomorrow's dinner — again,
roast beef, mashed potatoes, and a vegetable. She didn't care for the
second entree choice — ham sandwich. "Sorry, Jeeeerry!" 🛁 🛁

Personal: Jeremy and Colton are in their back yard, shooting their
bows and arrows and walking through the woods. They have a
great time together and are great friends. She didn't mention about
us coming back to visit her tomorrow because she doesn't know
what the doctors have planned.

6:40 p.m. @ RPCI

Debra was able to eat turkey, mashed potatoes and cake for dinner.
The doctor reported, "It's not quite right, Debra, there may an

infection in your port." She was scheduled for the surgery. Her foley was taken out. She's been walking now and the heart monitor was taken off. "Whew, Mom, progress!" ⬆

Personal: A group of them — Lisa and company — were going to the cabin this weekend, but trip was cancelled because of Lisa's cough. Later, Deb talked to Jeremy and he was in the back yard shooting his bow and arrows.

10/28/11, Fri. @ RPCI

Personal: Jeremy called Debra; the school sent him home — he has poison ivy! He probably caught it when he and Colton walked through the woods. A month ago, Colton had it all over, and they can't pinpoint the location. It's on Jeremy hands and face so he probably rubbed it on his clothes and when he took them off, that's were he got it. His father will be home around 6:00 and can call a pharmacist.

Later, Debra called and said Phil is taking Jeremy to a doctor today. "Mom, I feel so helpless just laying here. I should have my son with me. I should be the one who watches out for him, protects him, and does all the special, caring things for him." She was crying. ♀

7:30 p.m. @ RPCI

Debra, have you talked to Jeremy yet? "Not yet, Mom. Lisa is going to come and get him; all I want to do is go home and sleep. Dr. LaiLai told me he's not going to do any treatments for one month, but then said "I'll see you on Monday." (*What? Monday? Why?*) She doesn't know what that's about. He had already walked out before she could question him. Deb didn't ask him if he had the results of the MRI they took or maybe only a CT scan is what shows. She said: "Don't doctors realize when they surprise you by coming in your room and you're half asleep or watching TV, it takes a minute to put your brain in gear, but they make a simple statement and then walk out? It is so frustrating! And I lay here with all the questions in my mind, grrr!"

10/26/11, Wed. @ RPCI

The doctor gave Debra steroids — no cream. She was discharged.

Personal: "Mom, I don't know if I'm going to be up to going for the pumpkins on Saturday for Jeremy. He'll be disappointed." *"No, he won't be disappointed, Debra. We will offer to take him if he wants to go.*

It snowed today when Jerr and I were at Eastern Hills Mall, It is freezing and cold. We are very uncomfortable and can't wrap up enough to be warm. It must be the change in blood from our stays in Florida!

10/27/11, Thurs. - 8:00 p.m. —

Debra's in bed, not quite feeling well, yesterday wasn't well either. She started to get jerks in her arms and legs and almost went to hospital, but she fell asleep and when she woke up, the symptoms had alleviated a lot. She's still wobbly; Lisa walked her to the bathroom and kitchen, she hasn't wanted to eat very much.

"Sweetheart, we have a case of Ensure — or the Walgreen's brand that you prefer, and we can bring it over." She said she wants to get together sometime this weekend or early next week.

"Mom, it's so cold; Jerr gets sick in the cold weather. I was thinking, when are you going to Florida?"

"Sweetheart, we don't know; we don't want to yet; we'll see." "Why? Why? Is it because of me? You should have already left! Is it because of me?" (upset and panicking)

10/25/11, Tues., 11:00 a.m. —

Called Lisa to find out what was going on with Debra's phone again. She said, "I don't know, she has it with her." We made arrangements to meet at 3:00 p.m. at the half-way point.

At the arranged meeting place, we waited for 20 minutes, then called Lisa again. Debra answered Lisa's phone. We didn't like how she sounded, but she said she and Lisa will meet us. Much later after waiting another thirty minutes, Lisa drove out by herself, and we transferred all the food — freezer, refrigerator, canned goods — from our car to hers in the event we decided to leave for Florida.

Then in the parking lot, Lisa said she was going to call RPCI tomorrow because she felt Debra was lethargic and a bit disoriented, and sleeping too much. She said, "You're welcome to come to our house and see her to get another opinion and make sure I'm not making a lot out of nothing." Now we were very concerned.

Right from the parking lot, we called RPCI (Charron) immediately. We actually reached her! Charron stated that with Debra's "symptoms", she should be seen immediately at a local hospital and asked us what had Hospice said? We said, "HOSPICE??? What do you mean Hospice?" She replied that, "Debra was sent home to call Hospice." "I said absolutely not — not that I'm aware of! This is the first we've heard about Hospice. Why? I've seen her discharge forms, nothing was said anything about Hospice." I turned to Lisa, "Lisa, do you know anything about Debra having to go to Hospice?" She replied, "No, I don't."

Charron told us to let her know what was happening with Debra; to call her the next morning and tell her.

Jerr and I followed Lisa to her house and found Debra lying on a mattress on the floor; she could hardly answer me; she looked white as a sheet; she was freezing although the room was quite warm and Debra had on several layers of thermals. I knew immediately there was a problem. I finally was able to get her up and dressed and at 4:00 p.m. drove her to the hospital.

4:00 p.m. @ E/R NFMMH —

We got a wheelchair to carry Debra from our car into the building. She was taken in immediately; we were not able to see her
until one hour later. We were told she had pneumonia and her
red blood cells barely registered 6! She could barely speak to ask
for pain meds, which I did for her. She got upset when they tried
to give her the same story about taking Lortab every six hours,
saying she has always been given Dilaudid and then Lyrica 75 mg
for the pain in her back. "After all this time, don't my records show
that? Why do I have to fight every time for the same treatment?
I'm sorry I'm saying this to you, but honestly!" Her nurse, Eve,
had to start another IV line in her hand to give her the pain meds.
And when the first nurse came back and started her IV in the port,
she said it had really hurt with her pushing and shoving real deep.
Debra was crying. Was this payback for what she had said to them?
We were so frustrated! Must be why they don't let family into the
E/R initially?

7:00 p.m. In the ICU —

Debra's room is right next to an elevator and every cart and
wheelchair scraped over the floor bars. She was trying to sleep.
The staff was so loud and inconsiderate of people. There was
a group of three girls (nurses?) in a room in the back of E/R,
laughing and making fun of some of the people there. They could
be heard throughout the floor. I walked back there looking for
a public restroom; they just looked at me and kept on with their
raucous conversation.

7:30 p.m. —

Debra has been transferred out of ICU into a regular room where
it's finally very quiet, and she has been able to get her rest. She was
sounding much better to us, has been given three bags of blood;
was still on some kind of antibiotic called Vancoled IV*. We were
able to have a good conversation.

About midnight, Deb was given a turkey dinner. We stayed with her until 1:30 a.m. She said she was fed, was getting pain meds and was getting sleepy. "Please go home, guys, it's time for your dinner." She had no idea of the time. *"We love you, Debra."* "I love you two, too." 🛏️🛏️

When we returned home, I sobbed and sobbed, not only about her condition, about the treatment at the hospital and because of the condition of her room at Lisa's. About the hospital, I wanted to go in there and wipe the floors up with everybody who was so rude! I wanted to write letters to the hospital head. I wanted to write letters to the newspapers or call the TV stations. I wanted to go in, rip all the IVs out and take her in my arms and run somewhere she would be protected or to another hospital — a hospital where she would get excellent care — did they not know her condition, did they just not care? If there was a police who could help patients or parents in a hospital, I would have called them in a minute, but unfortunately, there isn't. Instead, we fell exhausted into sleep on top of the bed.

10/29/11, Sun. —

The next day we didn't wake up until 10:00 a.m. I waited until after breakfast to call Lisa and tell her what was happening with Debra. She was horrified. She asked us, "Is Debbie mad at me?" *"No, Lisa, Why?* " "Because I brought you guys to my house."

I said, *"Please don't be offended, Lisa, but Debra has to get off the floor. People walk into a house from the outside and there are bacteria and germs on their shoes and even more so with two dogs; they walk into bird or animal droppings, and Debra is sleeping on the floor breathing in all this stuff. No wonder she's had one infection after another."*

Lisa said that the dogs are very clean and there was a bed frame for Debra's mattress but she didn't want it.

I said, *"Well, she's no longer a teenager to camp out. Even though she's a* woman, she's still my little girl and she has cancer and she has to get off the floor. If there's not a bed frame, let us know, and we'll go out and get one. If she doesn't have sheets or blankets or a bedspread, we'll get those, too. Lisa, I know it's not your fault that she has another infection. And I know you haven't been well either. But let's improve Debra's living conditions. We'll help." Lisa said, "No, all the bedding was on the chair in her room after being laundered, but Debra didn't want to get up to have her bed changed." (OK, so we must have walked in on an unusual situation, which happens. We could understand Debra's condition and other issues.)

10/30/11, Sun., 9:30 a.m. @ NFMMH

Debra in ICU and not ready to go home, blood transfusions were finished. She was given some kind of sandwich after midnight when she was feeling nauseated, and she had been itching and scratching her skin. When Debra called the nurse, she didn't come. After another thirty minutes, Debra called for the nurse again, told her that she was nauseated and felt like throwing up. The nurse still didn't come. When she finally came, Deb could barely get the words out that she needed a tray when she threw up, so now there was a time-consuming cleanup and an irritated person. She was freezing and when she gets that feeling, she always throws up. She said, "You know, I try not to bother the nurses until I really need them." *Really, sweetheart!*

She talked about her living conditions at Lisa's and started crying. "Mom, I'm so embarrassed that you and Jerr saw me like that. That room never looks like you saw it nor does the house look like a shit hole. It made me feel like I would be the kind of person that would live in such conditions. I'm just sorry you had to see me, Mummy, you and Jerr. OMG. Even though it's far for you to come and see me at Lisa's, I just didn't really care. I couldn't even care. I was so sick. But it's easier to use the mattress on the floor because I don't think I can get up on a regular bed with my legs so weak." *"I'm so sorry, sweetheart. We needed to see you."* I told her of my talk with Lisa and buying the bed frame, and she was OK with that. She's also going to have a talk with Lisa when she gets out of the hospital, just the two of them.

10/31/11, Sun. —

Talked to Debra in the evening; she was very tired and had been sleeping a lot.

Personal: Jeremy and Colton were installing carpeting in Colton's bedroom. Then on Saturday, Jeremy was installing a wood floor in Lisa's hallway. "Mom, he's really proud of his skills in being able to complete these two projects

11:30 a.m. —

Debra is lying in bed; her legs are trembly, and she's still dizzy. The chemicals are still in her body; her urine is still coming out green.

"Debra, that's a strange one, and it's something I couldn't research; couldn't find it anywhere!" We were laughing and she said, "Not even under 'green peepee'?" 😂😂

(I tried calling RPCI, left messages on voice mails — no answer.)

10/31/11. Mon. —

No contact with Debra; phone keeps going into an immediate beep-beep-beep. Lisa does not answer her phone or call us back.

11/1/11, Tues. —

Debra is feeling better. She asked why were we still here? She said, "You don't have to wait for me, Mom, I'll be OK. Please leave for Florida. Don't put that burden on my shoulders, too. I have enough to deal with." Debra is discharged.

11/3/11, Thurs. —

She was feeling OK, just a bit tired but had been for walks around the neighborhood with the dogs. Tomorrow she's going with her father to Factory Outlet to look at bed frames. She's waiting for her meds to be delivered, then will go to the drugstore for a digital thermometer; the doctor said she needed to check her temperature every day. When it started to go up, she needs to get to the hospital sooner. Lisa said she had a blood pressure cuff and takes Debra's pressure every day and now will record the temperature. She has a calendar in Debra's room. What a truly precious friend.

11/8/11, Tuesday —

We had dinner at the Olive Garden — one of their specials.

Upstate delivers Lyrica 75 mg, Fluconazole 200 mg, Cefpodoxime* 200 mg.

11/9/11, Fri.

"Jerrrrry, happy birthday, you, big guy, you. I hope you have a wonderful day and be happy. I love you." "My sweetheart, I love you, too. Be well and let's take care of you." "Let's take care of all of us."

11/14/11, Mon. —

We sent a certified package to RPCI requesting Debra's CT scans and the 6/28 blood test. (*Never received — why? What are they hiding?*)

11/17/11, Thurs., 4:00 p.m. —

RPCI called Debra for an 11:00 a.m. appointment at the Amherst Clinic to see Dr. LaiLai. Lisa took her, and they sat there until 3:30 p.m. They watched everyone else come in, be treated and leave, and they still sat there. Finally, Dr. LaiLai (and Charron) called Debra in; Lisa went with her. Dr. LaiLai asked her how she was feeling. Deb told him "OK, except for what happened while I was in the hospital the last time."

He then told her, "Well, there's nothing else I can do for you. I'm not going to continue treating you." Debra sat for a few minutes, shocked. Then asked, "Why?"

He explained, The tiny little spot at the tip of her lung was now numerous spots like salt and pepper sprinkled all over and that he'd probably kill her with the chemo treatments before the cancer did! He told her to call Hospice. He walked out. (Her diagnosis is cervical cancer in her lungs — not lung cancer.)

Debra and Lisa were stunned and puzzled — what did he mean? On their way out, his secretary, Charron, whispered to Debra, "If it were me, I'd get a second opinion. You can get a second opinion." *(Now they say this? Why not in 2009? Or 2010? Or 2011?)*

All the doctors at other hospitals told Debra her lungs were clear and that they don't know why she keeps getting pneumonia, yet she doesn't have breathing problems. Upon examination, she is able to take a big, deep breath. At other hospitals, X-rays, CT scans say her lungs are clear. She felt Dr. LaiLai and Charron were so heartless and that she never believed him. What about the damage done to her heart? What about all the uncontrollable jerks on her arms and legs? He is the one who caused that. Lisa asked Charron, "What will Hospice do? Will they test her blood and tell her what meds to take? Charron said: "It doesn't matter."

I had so many questions. Debra was crying and crying with me, but not about herself, but about Jeremy. She said, "I don't want to destroy his life, Mummy; I want to see him graduate and see him admitted to the Police Academy as he wants. Last year, when I finally told him about my cancer, it interfered with his school work and his grades dropped for a while. This year, he's much better and he knows that entrance into the Academy depends on his grades. Now he's in Political Science as a prelude to the Academy and he loves his classes. I don't want to tell him anything because I don't know WHAT to tell him."

"Debra, we'll take you to your primary doctor, and he'll have to give you a referral to another oncologist. We'll get that second opinion." Debra told me she didn't have a primary doctor, but that she could go to the same doctor that Donna went to at Summit instead of the Family Medical on 10th Street.

After sobbing with her, I put the phone down and went and threw up in the bathroom and had diarrhea. I was shaking. (*Please, God, please, God, help us help Debra. Our strength comes from You.*)

Then I called her back. *"Debra, sweetheart, everything will be OK, we'll work it out, and we will get that second opinion. I'll call our oncologist friend tomorrow and get that reference to the new cancer treatment center that treats with laser and is in his own building. The one I've been telling you about all summer. We will work this out and we'll do whatever we can. And about Jeremy, you need to do what you are comfortable with — he's a great kid, but we understand about affecting his school work."*

All year, I had given Debra the newspaper clippings of the half-page ad from a new clinic in our area called CCS Oncology, about one mile from us in Williamsville. However, at the time, she felt uncomfortable changing to another clinic because she was so tied into RPCI and Dr. LaiLai, "Mom, I didn't want to start all over again with test after test and explanation after explanation." *"Debra, what we want for you is the best and a reason for hope. But yours is the final decision in your treatment and we respect that."*

I asked to talk to Lisa, and she then elaborated on what had been said because Debra probably didn't remember. They had stared at them, "What are they saying?" RPCI will Debra put on the Niagara Hospice list and they will help with her pain. They asked, "What's going to change in her life, why they can't operate?" She said Dr. LaiLai told her that it is cervical cancer that moved from that area to her lungs; it was not lung cancer and therefore she could not be referred to a lung specialist. (*After all this time, we're informed about this? Why haven't they done a PET scan*? Why not in all this time?*) Lisa and Debra are going to go to Hospice ahead of the time of her appointment and get information. She said Lisa hugged her and they cried together.

I told Lisa that Debra doesn't want to tell Jeremy yet. Lisa feels she should tell him because he may resent that everybody knew and didn't tell him. I told Lisa, "Well Debra feels like there's nothing to tell him right now. Wait until she's given more information." She said, "I guess you're right." (*Dear God, let this be the right decision.*) I asked Lisa, "Did they give her a 'time'?" She said, "No, nothing."

"Well, that gives me hope because RPCI is known for telling patients the truth, and they do give you a time frame. The fact that they haven't done so means that there's hope. Why can't we/she talk to someone? Why is there no one to help us? Why is there no information coming from the so-called experts?"

One day while Debra was staying with us, we saw a TV commercial about Cancer Treatment Centers of America. Jerr offered to take her there, and she could speak with them. She thought about it for a moment, went into her room and after a few minutes came out, and finally said, "If anything happens, I want to be home. I want to be near Jeremy. I want to be near where he can get to me." Jerr told her, "We'll take you anywhere you want, Debra, but please rethink what RPCI is doing to you -- or not doing for you."

I called Cancer Treatment Centers, learned the closest one to us was Philadelphia, and asked what we needed to do for our daughter, The man answered, "You've just done it. All it takes is a phone call and we take over from there. We'll make your travel arrangements, pick you up at the airport, transport you to our hotel and get you from the hotel to the Center. There Debra will meet with her treatment team, who will be the same group of people that will stay with her/you throughout her treatment. She will not have strange doctors coming and going in her room and having to repeat her symptoms over and over." I told him we would discuss it with Debra and let him know.

Personal: Debra said that Doug and Lisa will remove the chair and sofa from her room. Debra told us, "You should have seen this room when I moved in, Mom. It was used as a storage room. There was even a grill and crock pot in there. I told Lisa, 'I could cook my own meals in my room, just throw in some food and all I needed to do is go out to take a shower.' *"Debra, you can have a garden hose connected through the window and then you wouldn't even have to do that."* She said, "Boy, I can just see that, Mom." We were laughing about the concept! 😂😂

Then she said, "Mom, please call Charron and tell her 'my daughter called me in tears' and find out what she says."

Personal: Debra said Donna spent a few minutes with her, then her father took them to the Park Avenue Coat Company to get a warm jacket for Jeremy, and ended up getting Donna two shear jackets. Debra selected a winter jacket, a furry one that looked designer-like, but it's real warm, it looks like the jackets they wear on the Housewives of New Jersey. *(Who?)*

I asked if there was a Bed, Bath & Beyond nearby to Lisa's house? She said, "Yes, there's one near the Boulevard Mall." Debra told me she had gone to Wal-Mart and had seen a bed sheet set (Joe Boxer) that she really liked. "Mom, probably for the kids returning to dorms!" I told her, "Debra, fix your room up real nice like you always do with your apartments."

"Mom, after I know what kind of treatment I'm going to get, we will get everything organized. I put the Christmas crib in the fake fireplace here in my room and have my warm clothes in a little dresser. But I remember the beautiful Christmas trees you always had in our house and I tried to do mine like yours. And all the presents wrapped and piled under the tree — OMG. Then you went from our own Christmas tree to getting one for the City and from that Christmas tree gathering came the fabulous Festival of Lights. Awesome."

"Debra, I will call Jerr's oncologist tomorrow and ask him about that treatment center in Williamsville; will write a certified letter for you to send RPCI again asking for your records especially the one from 6/28." She promised to call Social Security to see about her claim. I told her I would call her tomorrow. *"We love you, Debra."* "I love you two, too."

Lisa told me Debra's father and Donna walked Debra up and down the driveway.

Lisa called Charron and asked why a blood panel hadn't been done to monitor her A1C, etc. Charron said, "It's the disease." *(and.....???)*

11/18/11, Fri. — Telecon with Charron @ RPCI, 3:30 p.m. —

The conversation follows:

Lorr.: Charron, this is Lorraine, Debra's mother, can you please tell me what happened yesterday? She called me hysterical, in tears and said Dr. LaiLai told her there was nothing further he can do for her and wasn't going to treating her any more and walked out of the room. What does that mean?

S: No, Dr. LaiLai had no other options for treating Debra, he had exhausted all options, and he had no more treatment options for this disease. We are an Institute and according to the ESCO (sp?) guidelines, he had reached the maximum treatment. *(Upon researching ESCO, the only reference I found is listed below — does that mean Debra was being used as an experiment? Is that why no medical records were ever given to her? OMG!)*

L: *Why couldn't she have been referred to a lung specialist at RPCI instead of just putting her out on the street? I went on the Internet last night and what came up for lung cancer was RPCI.*

S: She doesn't have lung cancer; she has cervical cancer which has spread to her lung and chest — metastasis which the chemo does not touch. Dr. LaiLai told her he would probably kill her with the chemo before the cancer did.

L: So, are you saying she's going to die?

S: No, not at all. Just that Dr. LaiLai, in his defense, has exhausted all options according to the "guidelines". Further treatment may be possible outside the Institute. I suggested this to her — that if it were me, I would seek a second opinion. Dr. LaiLai had Debra admitted as in-patient for this chemo. If this isn't treated, then it may become a problem.

L: RPCI has always been known for palliative, compassionate care, and we haven't found this to be true.

S: I'm sorry you feel that way.

L: Well, I do because after being given this news, there was no one to counsel her or help her accept this news. She was just left to walk out, carrying the news with her.

S: Amherst is only a satellite clinic and not fully staffed with a social worker or a psychologist.

L: Then why is bad news being given there? Her appointment was 11:00 a.m. and she sat there until 3:30 p.m. How can people be treated like this? Then why have her go to Amherst in the first place?

S: No, Dr. LaiLai left at 1:20 p.m.; we weren't behind on that day. She was seen before that. Debra has been offered the services of a psychologist for coping mechanism on her disease. (*Debra said not true about the offer, and oh yes, she and Lisa sat there until 3:30 p.m.. Everyone in the clinic was talking about schedules being behind and everybody was a bit frustrated.*)

L: Debra has never, ever told me that this counseling was offered. (*Debra does not recall the service of a psychologist being offered to her.*)

S: Debra seemed fine when she left the clinic. All she said was she was going to call her Mom and she left.

L: How would you feel hearing this news and then being put out on the street? A person can't think. She and I feel it was very callous and heartless how she was told, and Dr. LaiLai just walking out of the room.

S: There were many times that she missed her appointments and never called in (*Not so; I have the records*).

L: Those were probably some of the times she wasn't informed of an appointment, or she was in a hospital. We have the schedules and the errors in scheduling and cancellations. I know she only missed two appointments. On another subject, Debra and I have requested a copy of her CT scans four times. We've also requested the blood test results from 6/28/11, when she was told her blood chemistry was OK and later that night, she ended up in a hospital with a count of 4 and a mild heart attack.

S: We don't have anything to do about that. I can give you a phone number to Medical Reports and you can request them there. Is there anything more I can do? I will do what I can here to help Debra. (*Such a fake, flat monotone of voice.*)

L: I'm sure she doesn't want to have anything more to do with RPCI.

Another call to RPCI Medical Records, one girl I spoke to couldn't find her signed Release and referred me to another person. All he found was that a Field Analyst from Social Security had come to the hospital on 10/3/11 and spent hours copying her medical records. (Really?! *OMG, does that mean there's movement on her case, and she may be close to receiving a decision? Praise the Lord!*) RPCI emailed me another Release Form for more copies, and I mailed them to Debra to send to RPCI. (*What was unbelievable to me was that Medical Records were departments within RPCI, and the doctors could not provide the records that Debra kept requesting? And signing all these Release Forms — was that just a delay tactic — or mismanagement?*)

I also emailed CCS Oncology in Williamsville requesting the earliest consultation and/or treatment for Debra. A message appeared on my screen which stated that emails would be replied to within 1-2 business days.

I called our oncologist friend and asked for the referral to a gynecological oncologist in Williamsville. His secretary informed us the doctor was off that afternoon and weekend and that the message was in the computer, and he would get it on Monday. She also gave us the information for the doctors at the new clinic. I called and requested an appointment for Debra.

When I gave Debra all this news, she said, "Well, why didn't Dr. LaiLai explain that? Why couldn't he refer me to someone that he knew could treat me? And what about the uncontrollable jerks and spasms of my hands and feet — did they say anything about that? Are they permanent? Well, they haven't heard the last of me yet. I'll go to a lawyer if I have to. I've been mistreated — not only emotionally but physically."

We sent a letter to RPCI requesting a copy of the CT scans and the blood test. (*Never received.*)

11/21/11, Mon. —

In two days, Debra had an appointment with Dr. Yi, Wednesday, 11/30/11 at 1:30 p.m. I gave Debra the update about CCS. May at CCS will send Debra a Release Form to obtain her records from RPCI (*good luck*). Debra may have to get her own oncologist. (*Again, something Debra hadn't wanted to make a change.*)

Personal: Jeremy wasn't with her this weekend; he went hunting with his father. All she's going to tell him right now is that she's changing doctors and going somewhere else for her treatment. She sees her own pain management doctor on 12/7/11 She said "Thank you, Mummy". (*Thank God!!*)

11/24/11, Thanksgiving Thurs. —

Debra called for my birthday! 📤 She, Donna and Jeremy had planned to have a little Thanksgiving dinner together. She was not feeling well; she was very cold and could not get warm. I reminded her that this was the way she felt last time when her red blood cells were dangerously low and to keep an eye on her symptoms. Later that afternoon, Lisa called 911 and Debra went to MSMH.

(Donna's version: Four months later on 3/15/12, Donna told me that she was the one who called 911; she went with Debra. Lisa volunteers at soup kitchen and shelter. Lisa must have done the shopping and she bought fresh yams for my special 'puff' dish. Donna found that the oven was turned off and the turkey wasn't cooking and had to be reset but it was only off one hour. Donna cooked all the food but Debra was too sick to check on it. When she went to the hospital, Donna had to drive from Niagara Falls to Buffalo to pick Jeremy up. Jeremy and Donna never had their Thanksgiving dinner until 11:00 p.m. and by the time they got back to Lisa's everybody was back home and some of the food had been thrown away.)

11/26/11, Sat. @ MSMH, 3rd floor — ("Happy Birthday, Donna!)

Debra was admitted, diagnosed with pneumonia again. She said. "I didn't even get a chance to have Thanksgiving dinner and be with Jeremy. Is this going to happen every weekend he's there?", she asked. "I complained all the way to the hospital that I did not want to go but I could not breathe. Other than that, I feel good but haven't eaten in two days. The doctor here asked me what treatment I am going to have now that RPCI isn't treating me. I told him I had an appointment with Dr. Yi and he nodded his head and smiled. Maybe I can have an oncologist here in Niagara Falls."

Later, I kept calling Debra's room and there was no answer. I then called the 3rd Floor nurses station and she found the phone wasn't working; the aide brought another phone to Debra, and we had our usual long conversation.

11/27/11, Sun. @ MSMH —

"Mummy, yesterday my doctors (Dr. Shaw / Dr. Shenk?) thought I had pneumonia, but I do not. There's an infection somewhere; thought it was in my port, but it is not. I'm being given antibiotics, magnesium and potassium. Blood chemistry was low but not as low as before but I am being given blood transfusions again. The reason I had not eaten in three days and had no appetite, nothing appealed to me and I could not even drink anything was I was slightly dehydrated, as usual it seems. My ulcer is acting up. Nothing has been said about my electrolytes this time, but you found that low electrolytes affect my legs and that is why I cannot walk, which is so annoying — you take two steps and you can't stand up. I see why people get so frustrated and short-tempered; it's awful, Mom. There's so much that I want to do.

"The assistant oncologist came to see me and said that immediately upon my discharge, I was to go to their office; I don't need an appointment. She's putting in my record that I will be a "walk-in". I will see how comfortable I am with the oncologist, and apparently, he is receiving new patients. This doctor said I have to be treated immediately. At least it will be in Niagara Falls. Mom, I told her, 'One thing I do not want is the same anesthetic I was given the last time — twilight sleep — it caused a problem for three days.' She agreed. This new oncologist is on Military Road and is the one who discovered the cure for Lou Garrick's disease. There's hope again, Mom.

"Maybe the reason Dr. LaiLai couldn't treat me anymore was

because I was in Phase 3 - the 3rd year - does that mean Medicaid wouldn't let him treat me, maybe the first year is Phase 1, then the 2nd year is Phase 2 and now I'm going into Phase 3? I don't know but why didn't he tell me that was the reason? Do I start all over again with this new doctor? Why have I not been given the information I need, it's so frustrating, Mom."

Afternoon: "Mom, the doctor said the blood culture indicated the infection was in the area of the port; so all the infections must have been coming from the port. It is being removed tomorrow. I will have to decide where to put in another port but I need to make it to my Wednesday appointment with Dr. Yi. The woman who answered the phone at OCC told me just let them know. (*Yes, a human being actually answering the phone! She was extremely nice.*) "What a change, Mom!"

Debra finally was able to eat chicken breast, potatoes, today she is being given more solid food.

Personal: Debra did not answer cell phone. Someone put in the closet, and she didn't want to get up and get it. I called into her room. She requested the package and sent the certified mail to RPCI requesting the CT records and blood test of 6/28. She should receive the package with the medical chronology tomorrow. She hopes to be discharged in time to go to see Dr. Yi. "I should be OK, Mummy."

Personal: Yesterday Doug and Colton took Jeremy hunting all day; Doug caught a button buck. (OMG!) Then last night after 10:00, Jeremy called her and said they were at Jocco's eating pizza subs! "Here I am worrying about him getting home with everybody in the hospital, and getting something to eat, whether he's sleeping in my bed, and they are out having a good time! GOOD! I'm happy!"

11/28/11, Mon. @ MSMH —

Spiritual care was administered today.

Doctors are going to take the port out some time this afternoon. She again told the doctors, "I do not want the same anesthetic I was given before at RPCI." She was given a total of two bags of blood transfusion; still being given antibiotics; no more vitamins.

7:30 p.m. —

She's so tired and sleepy. The port was removed this afternoon about 4:00 p.m.; she doesn't remember a thing, nor did she feel anything. The doctor said they did not use the same anesthetic as used before, but she doesn't know what was used. "Obviously, I did not have the same reaction, Mom."

The Sacrament of the Anointing of the Sick was administered to Debra! (*A fact I did not learn until 11/6/12! Why? Why? Why? Was it felt this was necessary? The decision to take this step is not taken lightly, but why? It was always believed that this Sacrament was administered to the dying, but recently it is given for other reasons.*)

In the Catholic faith, until recent years, the sacrament was called *last rites* because it was usually administered when the person receiving the sacrament was in grave danger of dying. The term is sometimes more broadly used to refer to the reception of all of the Last Sacraments— Confession, Holy Communion, and the Anointing of the Sick. Last Rites is another term, very common in past centuries but rarely used today, for one of the seven sacraments of Catholics, the Sacrament of the Anointing of the Sick, which is administered both to the dying and to those who are gravely ill or are about to undergo a serious operation, for the recovery of their health and for spiritual strength.

11/29/11, Tues. —

Debra was supposed to have an appointment with her dentist, Dr. Sachdeva, but unfortunately, it had to be cancelled. The doctor told her that it was "OK, Debra, just call when you're able to come in."

We purchased their airline tickets for Jeremy's spring break

— depending on what Dr. Yi says about Debra being able to travel and how she feels, however, she was so happy when we told her the schedule. "Wow, Mom, something for me and Jeremy to look forward to. I can hardly wait!"

11/29/11, Tues., 11:00 a.m. @ MSMH —

Debra said the area where they took the port out really hurts and is sore; pain meds do not help it. She's not being given any anti-biotics, blood, or vitamins. "I don't know if I am going to be discharged in time to meet the 11/30 appt with CCS. Mom, will you change the appointment for me and tell them why?"

Later, Debra called CCS herself and her appointment was changed to Monday, 12/5/11, 11:00 a.m. per Mandy who asked her, "Were you sent a New Patient packet?" She answered, "I do not know because my Mom called on Tuesday and I came to the hospital on Thursday."

"Mom, I also have a 12/7 appointment with my pain med doctor just to pick up the prescription."

7:00 p.m.

I called Debra's room but she didn't answer the phone. I called the nurses' station, she said she was probably in a deep sleep (No, Debra said, she was in the bathroom.) She feels sick, her stomach hurts, I asked if she had been able to eat? "Yes." "Debra, tell the nurse about the stomach, you're being given your meds including Prilosec, but it could be a symptom of something else." None of the doctors have been in to see her yet, and no one has said anything about her being discharged.

11/30/11, Mon., 2:00 p.m. —

"Mom, I'm waiting to get discharged; everything feels OK, yeaah! My chest doesn't hurt any more. No doctors have come in yet, but

I'll wait and see what the discharge slip says." Debra was finally discharged and then told me it's snowing lightly — yukky.

12/5/11, Mon., 1:00 a.m. —

Debra's appointment with Dr. Yi at CCS Oncology was 25 minutes long! She and Lisa had just returned home at 3:30 p.m., because Lisa had a couple other errands to run. She really likes Dr. Yi; he was shocked especially after seeing her medical reports; he asked her, "Why after one year did you not seek a second opinion?" He's so disgusted about her treatment, just kept shaking his head. (*As I've been speaking about Debra's treatment everywhere I go, we've also now been told by others that Dr. LaiLai and RPCI is "old school" and do not believe in the new technology.*) CCS use pinpoint radiation. Every Friday, the patient is given a printed weekly report. Dr. Yi immediately ordered a PET scan on Thursday, 12/8/11 and then he will discuss treatment with Debra on Monday, 12/12/11. (*Dr. LaiLai has too many patients and many of them end up coming to CCS for treatment.*)

I talked to Lisa who also felt very comfortable with Dr. Yi. He took a lot of time with Debra almost 20-25 minutes, leaving the room twice, once for two minutes to tell his secretary to schedule Debra for the PET scan and then to get the medical reports from RPCI which were faxed over to him immediately! (*Really!*) He's restaging her treatment, the PET scan will show the hot spots, and then he'll set up a new program.

"Mom, when I had the port removed, it was the same surgeon who did the skin tags on my neck, and I reminded him of that saying. "You know when you removed my two skin tags......with a paper cutter!" We were laughing. However, he also said, "Whoever did the port really did a good job, I could hardly pull it out." Debra couldn't feel any pain or anything during the procedure, but the pulling was yucky. (*My knees and stomach felt queasy!*) "Mom, do you remember that I kept saying I don't feel like I have anything wrong with me? I wonder if it's true!" (*Please, Jesus, let it be true and protect my daughter. Show mercy to her on this road she is traveling. Bless these new doctors and this new clinic.*)

Personal: "Mummy, I had a wonderful gift today. Jeremy and I went shopping on Saturday as he had a lot of gift cards for his birthday. We went to lots of stores at the Boulevard Mall and had a real good time. When I got tired walking, he let me hold on to his arm as we walked along.

"Then on Sunday, Jeremy's cheeks and ears were red and he finally told me, 'My ear really hurts, Mom, it has so much pain.' I called Phil to inform him before we went to the clinic. His medical card was OK and I could sign as his parent." Debra immediately took him to a clinic on Niagara Falls Blvd. and they sat there for three hours, they were so busy with lots of people in for sore throats, etc. The doctor took a swab of his throat and then looked at his ear and said, "Oh, boy, do you have an ear infection!" The swab on his throat also revealed tonsillitis but not serious enough to have them taken out. He was given antibiotics and within one hour, he was already feeling better. He had suffered for two days with this pain and his grandfather didn't do anything for him. "Oh, Mommy, I wish I could protect Jeremy from all harm and from all pain. But do you remember how you cringed about us getting our shots and you sprayed our butts or thighs with medication for burns, and we never felt anything? Even with the huge needles they had in those days! You still do that to yourself and Jerr just for blood tests!"

Personal: Chris is bringing her pile of mail over and Debra hopes there's a notice from Social Security.

12/7/11, Wed., 11:15 a.m. — Debra's call

Good news! Social Security has finally approved her disability claim — Hallelujah! She won't get $836 as she had thought because child support is deducted and sent to Phil. "But that's OK, Mom, I will do anything for Jeremy. I'm so happy!" She was worried about the child support piling up, but it is something tolerable. Sh sh doesn't want anybody to know about it for now.

Her shoulder hurts; she's taking pain meds but they don't touch it; the stitches feel like they are pulling. Debra feels so foggy. "The oncologist who removed my port did not mention the insertion of another one. The nurse is the same one."

12/9/11, Fri. — Debra calls

A PET scan at CCS was done and she will have another consultation with Dr. Yi on Monday. "I just love them there, Mom. I've been given a gift — my humanity back! I'm a person, I'm a human being in pain, and I'm a name to them!"

12/11/11, Sun., 10:00 p.m. —

Debra has a slight temperature of 100°. She took it earlier this evening and now Lisa is taking it again. The concern is a possible infection or low red blood cells. She didn't even know why she decided to take her temperature; she was not dizzy, her eyes were kind of focusing funny and the jerking arms and legs were back. (*I really hope that is not permanent*.) Her arm is so sore that she can't raise it above her head, she doesn't know why. The pain in her back isn't as bad now.

Personal: There was blizzard on Friday, almost 4" of snow, and it's still on the ground. Donna called her on Friday and asked them to help her clear out her apartment, and then on Saturday, she asked Jeremy to move her bed. Deb didn't want him to do it by himself because of the back pain he has.

12/12/11, Mon. —

Dr. Yi informed Debra that the PET scan revealed the hot spots were in her stomach — two spots blocking her airway. She said everything she went through was for nothing?! ♀ We both said how much we hated Dr. LaiLai and RPCI and what they were not doing for her there. Why was a PET scan never done? Why was he giving her chemo for something that she didn't have? Dr. Yi never said anything about the lungs. He sent her for a blood test at Quest on Youngs and although they only take patients by appointment, when Debra walked in and quietly asked, "Could you please help me? My doctor needs to have this test ASAP." The girl took her immediately. Other women were complaining that they had appointments, had been waiting for 20 minutes, and they were fasting. The girl was stressed; apparently she was taking care of both the window and the lab. Once again, Debra said she was blessed by a gift. The doctor have her a prescription for antibiotics because she must have an infection, and he doesn't want to start treatment until that is cleared. She told Dr. Yi about the removal of the port and the pain that was now in her collarbone and right arm and that she can't even lift her arm above her head.

12/13/11, Tues. - 11:00 a.m. —

Debra is having another PET scan. Dr. Yi will evaluate it from a different perspective, and then he said he'll plan out a treatment for her. He'll see the hot spots and where the activity is and go from there.

3:00 p.m. —

"Mom, I made a mistake — oops. It was not a PET scan — it was Body Image Measurement. The technician takes a soft white blanket; it's like a body cast but doesn't harden, she tucked it around me; then went into a machine (like an MRI), it was spinning and had red lights; then it stopped and she opened my robe, put on a sticky circle and marked an X in red. These marks will stay there until next Tuesday. She marked the middle of my breast bone, then two other spots. I expected to be there for ten minutes but it took 1-1/2 hours. Another measurement will be done on Monday. Results of the blood test hasn't been received yet, so they couldn't give me the prescription for antibiotics, but my fever was coming down; it was 99° today. Dr. Yi starts the treatment on Tuesday."

Personal: Debra drove herself to CCS today as Lisa had another doctor appointment. Debra felt so good. Deb has offered Lisa money for gas, and she refused because Doug fills the cars with his business credit card as he owns the company.

12/15/11, Thurs. — @ MSMH

We called Debra's cell phone twice at home and there was no answer. I then called the hospitals patient information numbers and found out she's been admitted at MSMH and is in room #335, called there, but no answer. Will call again and then will call the nurse's station there. In the meantime, Lisa called and informed us Debra was in the hospital; not with stomach flu but now it's with a bowel obstruction* according to the doctors.

12/16/11, Fri. @ MSMH —

Debra has a bowel obstruction which was revealed with an x-ray and CT scan; she's had blood tests; she has a tube down her nose to her stomach (a very painful process!) with fluids trying to break up the obstruction. The doctor informed her, "If this doesn't help and it doesn't drain, I may have to do surgery which is standard procedure in cases like yours." Lisa said Debra was so pale yesterday, but when her vitals were taken on the way to hospital, her red blood cells are OK and everything else was OK. She has to poop in a bottle and she said "Yuk!" This pain in her stomach is very painful; they are giving her pain meds but right now, they don't help. Later, a surgeon came in and said, "Hopefully, this will break up on its own." "And, Mom, you'll never believe what he said caused this — CHEMO! I don't trust Dr. LaiLai, in my opinion, he lied to me. I have not eaten anything, just a few ice chips, this is worse than having the hysterectomy; I wouldn't wish this on anybody, not anybody. Mom, I had a dream that I walked into Roswell and was choking Dr. LaiLai by the throat!" *("You couldn't — I would have already done it, sweetheart!")*

The day nurses and aides are all very nice and helpful. The doctor now is doubling the pain meds. Debra also has a pain in her groin, like she pulled a muscle last week but said that if anything was there, it would have shown up on the PET scan.

(According to the information I found on WebMD* for a bowel obstruction, the food groups that she is supposed to eat to prevent the condition, she can't — brown rice, whole wheat pasta, vegetables, beans, peas, lentils, fruit.)

Debra asked me to call CCS and alert them that she may not make her Monday/Tuesday appointment. I spoke to May but never gave her my Florida phone number, but about an hour later, Dr. Yi called me and left a message. He said he was very concerned about Debra and that I could call him at any time of the day or night and gave us his personal cell phone number. He told me she's likely to recover enough to be discharged by Sunday, but if not, have her call and they will place her appointment at the top of the CCS priority list. He also said, *"The PET scan revealed abnormal outtake in proportion of the stomach but it's treatable." (Could this be the cancer acting up?)* I informed Deb.

She has had an argument with the night nurse who was falsely "nicey" and treating Debra like she doesn't know what should be done. "After two years of treatments and needles and hospitals, I know what should be done!" The nurse told Debra that she was a "super IV giver". "Mom, she wasn't, it took her four punctures — was this payback again because of my outburst, but I am in pain? Don't these people realize that after their rough treatment, it is also their words that are left with you, and you lay here thinking and crying? Why are they even here?"

12/17/11, Sat. —

We requested medical records from RPCI — the CT scans and blood results of 6/28/11. *(Never received.).*

12/17/11, Sat. —

I called Debra and she said, "Call me back later, Mom."

12:30 p.m. —

Debra said she was having an anxiety attack and called for the nurse. She cried, cried, and cried. She felt the tape was coming loose from her nose, and she could feel the tube scratching her throat. She was being taken for an X-ray and they couldn't take her down. She's very low in potassium and was told that would make her emotional. She's also low on oxygen and was being given that. She was still crying and crying. She told the nurse "I feel that because I'm not eating, I'm going to get sick." The nurse informed Debra that she was being hydrated. "I know, but in my mind, I'm going to get sick from not eating and that throws me in a tizzy." The nurse could not fix the tape and had to get somebody who knows what to do. "It's scratching my throat!"

Later she apologized to the nurse who said it was not necessary. "Mom, I've been passing gas, farting like crazy *(Good — I think?!)* The b/m is still green, looks like pond scum. I guess I should do what that TV doctor says, drink something like Liquid Plumber! All in all, it's been a very bad day. How do I relax, Mom? If this hospital can't help me, who can? Who?!"

"Debra, let's calm you down, close your eyes and picture all the parks you and Jeremy went to and walked among the trees, feeling the breeze, wading in the cool streams, crossing over the little bridges, and you told me that if you stood very quietly without speaking, you could hear the birds and see animals and deer and squirrels and how happy you both were and how you and Jeremy shared the love of nature.

"And then do you remember how when you girls were not feeling well, I would rub your back until you fell asleep. Do you remember all the good times we had and how you are now sharing these with your son, Jeremy, and he's so lucky to have such love from a mother, and....." Debra didn't answer me. I called out her name a couple of times, then hung up and tried calling her back and the line was ringing busy. In a panic, I called the nurses station, who went in to check on Debra and came back and told me that when she saw Debra was asleep, she picked up the phone and hung it up. Debra was asleep! "Is she OK, is she OK?" "Yes, she is, she's sleeping." (*Thank, God, and thank you Jesus for your gift of healing of my daughter. Please have your angels surround her and protect her.*) *Hours later, Debra called and said she had a wonderful sleep,* "Thank you, Mummy, thank you. I love you." *"We love you, too, sweetheart."*

5:30 p.m.-

Debra's being given blood transfusions, two bags and hopes it will give her strength, because she's so weak. She's being given anti-anxiety medicine plus the pain meds. Doctor came in to see her and she was crying. The anxiety meds will stop her flipping out at the drop of a hat. She's still in pain, but it comes and goes, stomach gets hard as a rock, then goes away. Her b/m is now brown but her urine is still green. She said she feels like an alien! She was given a throat spray for the pain.

She still hasn't had anything to eat but ice chips which gave her a stomach ache, so she's being given warm water instead to try. Now, she was laughing, and still joking with the nurses. One nurse was putting in the blood transfusion, the other one on the other side, and Debra said she feels like a diva with all the attention!

12/18/11, Sun. —

Debra is feeling somewhat better. The doctor never told her he was cutting off her pain medication, Dr Shake (?), she has pain still in her stomach and in her back. The weekend nurse, the same one as yesterday, was still arguing. She's lazy and doesn't answer the call bell. She said she can't believe Debra was given pain meds two hours before her discharge. Debra told her, "Well, I was. I always was!" The nurse asked that the doctor be paged to talk to her — nothing yet. If Debra is going to be miserable, she might as well be miserable at home where it's cozy warm, it's so cold in here.

"Later the doctor came with an attitude, a real asshole, Mom, excuse me! The nurse must have said something to him, because he came in and immediately said, real loud, 'I am not giving you IV pain meds, you are eating food now!'

"Doctor, I've always been given IV pain meds, even while I'm eating."

Doctor: Are you the doctor?

Debra: Is this vengeance? Just being given the Lortab pills, so I can lay here in pain. Why are you so mad at me? All I'm asking is for pain meds!

Nurse: You're not his only patient, you know!

"Debra, we've decided that we returning home. We have decided that we want to spend Christmas and Hanukah in Williamsville, and besides………."

"Please, Mom, no, you're not! Do you want to lay that guilt on me — what if something happens on the plane or the road. It's freezing here, what if Jerr gets sick? I'm fine; I'm being taken care of, and we talk every day or several times a day! That's the contact I want with you right now. I tell you everything the doctors tell me. Besides I'm going to be discharged shortly."

12/19/11, Mon. —

Debra was discharged about 5:30 p.m., Dr. Shaw (⚱) love him, told her to take potassium because it's low.

It's very cold outside; she doesn't have a coat because she came to hospital in ambulance and didn't have a chance to grab one, but Chris is bringing her a coat when he picks her up. She'll call me when she gets her cell phone charged.

I called Mandy at CCS and Jaime, the therapist, and made Debra's appointment with Dr. Yi for next Wednesday, 12/28/11, 10:30 a.m. He will have to do a CT simulation and then he'll determine the course of treatment.

Personal: "Mom, guess what — Jeremy wants one of those cameras that you put in the woods and it films if deer come by. Isn't that a neat thing — I never knew something like that existed. That will be his Christmas present."

12/20/11, Tues., 7:30 p.m. —

Debra was home but had a terrible stomach ache last night, and thought it was because she took the huge potassium pill and has had hardly anything to eat, but she feels better today. "Yeeah, Mummy! ⚓ ⚓

Personal: Chris brought over all her mail and lo and behold — there are a few envelopes from the Dept. of Treasury! She got her Social Security Disability checks going back to September! She will get a substantial amount every month less the child support for Jeremy. The last time she had any money was in 2009 when she got the small settlement from State Insurance Fund for the accident. Now she felt what a gift this money was — and at Christmas time, too! She was given a MasterCard Debit card from Social Security, and SSA will add the money automatically to that card, and she uses it like a credit card, no fees, no interest, no charges, no bank charges, just the money.

Personal: Debra's going to her pain management doctor tomorrow and then shopping for Jeremy. She wants to get all the shopping done in one day. Jeremy wants a pair of Reebok sneakers. "*Debra, get a picture of them from the newspaper and put it in an envelope and then later you can go shopping together for them."* He also wants to go to Los Angeles at some time in the future, but he loves Florida the best. Then she said she would be able to pay for their own airline tickets when they come to see us in the spring during his spring break. "Mom, what a pleasure it will be to pay our way." Maybe the two of them can stay a night at the Westin Diplomat (across the street from us)! "Won't that be a gift, Mom — we loved that place!" *(Oh, drat, now what do I give them for Christmas?!* ⚓ ⚓*)*

12/21/11 -Wed., 8:20 a.m. —

She just opened her envelopes from Dept. of Treasury; initially had put them aside; she was so excited just with the information she had just received. She had thought they were just notices about the deposit into her debit account, but they were the actual checks all of them in the thousands of dollars! It seems that she always thought she knew what her monthly benefit was going to be, she received almost seven months back benefits! She doesn't know what to do with the money! She doesn't want to open a bank account, she doesn't want to keep the cash around, she suggested perhaps sending me the largest checks and then she can save the money for Jeremy. We can open a joint account when we get there so that she can have access to the money whenever she wants. *"Debra, do not send the checks now — wait until after Christmas with the chaotic mail, and we'll talk again."*

12/22/11, Thurs. —

"Mom, I feel really good." We're having a wonderful time. I'm so excited about Christmas but it's so cold outside."

12/23/11, Friday —

No word from Debra. She doesn't answer my calls. I started calling the hospitals and they did not have her listed as a patient or in the E/R. *(Thank, God.)*

12/24/11, Sat. —

"Merry Christmas, sweetheart. My prayers tonight at Midnight Mass will continue to be for you and for Jeremy."

"I know, Mom. It will be a Merry Christmas and a great new year! Mom, do you remember the year when Donna and I kept pestering you for a "real" Christmas tree? (*Yes, groan.*) In our family room, our Christmas tree — although beautiful and full — it was an artificial one with branches you stick into a pole, but it looked spectacular when decorated. You left after dinner saying you'd be right back. Later, we all went to Midnight Mass and came home, Donna and I finally went to bed, hoping to hear bells and jingles on the roof. Years later, we learned that you had gone to a Christmas tree lot, asked the attendant if he would sell you two tops from the Christmas trees (*No, he didn't sell them, he gave them to me!*) You hid them in the trunk of the car. Then when you thought we were asleep, you took your needlework basket and with red yarn, tied a hundred bows on the tips of every branch and put a star at the top. You sat there for hours and had just gone to bed, when we woke up early in the morning to see if Santa Claus had come — and what did we find? We found next to our beds, our REAL trees! What a perfect gift! We kept those trees for years and years even after the needles had dried out. Years later, when we had left the house and you moved, guess what you found in our little storage space in our bedroom. Yup, our little Christmas tree tops! You told us you had to wear gloves because the branches had sharp needles, but the bows were still there — but we loved those trees; we loved you for the gift." *"Thank you, my sweetheart, for the gift of this memory!"* 🌲🌲

12/25/11, Sun. — A BLESSED AND HAPPY CHRISTMAS. We hope. (*Little did we know what lay ahead.*)

12/28/11, Wed.- 7:00 p.m.

Debra met with Dr. Yi; they did coordinates, put more markers on the side of her chest and breastbone. She starts treatments again on Tuesday and every day for three weeks, then he'll do another PET scan and see where she is. She will schedule the van to take her; Lisa can't go every day because of her own appointments, but she said it was no problem. "Mom, one elegant lady I met in the waiting room asked me if I had gotten the "mark of Zorro". (*The "mark of Zorro" she referred to were the markings on her body for the radiation treatments.*) They laughed, and Debra said, "Yes! I did." The lady told her, "I've received fifteen treatments and I'm now done!" Patients in the waiting room were so happy and upbeat and talking to each other. "My gosh, Mom, what a difference." Dr. Yi put Debra on steroids which would help with her breathing, her stomach pain, and something else, she didn't remember.

Personal: Lisa got on the phone and thanked us for the Bed, Bath & Beyond gift card for Christmas, and she said it would come in handy because their bed is so terrible, she wants to buy a foam mattress topper, and the gift card would go a long way in helping them with that. I told her about the BBB coupons I sent, you can use up to four of them if you buy four items and can use them at the same cash register; that's a great discount.

12/29/11, Thurs., 7:30 p.m. —

"Mummy, my immune system must be up because when I went to the doctor's office, everybody was coughing, sneezing, and I have not gotten sick! That was a first! Gosh, Mom, what a gift now at this new place. I feel so hopeful! And as I mentioned before everyone is super nice and the patients are so positive and happy. You know it makes you feel better without all the depressing people at RPCI with the blank, hopeless look in their faces. I love you, Mummy. You have given me so much. Thank you for getting me here." "*We love you too, sweetheart.*"

"My little Christmas tree in my room at Lisa's looks so cute; it has red ribbons and tiny ornaments and satin skirt. It reminds me again of our "real" Christmas tree surprise you gave me and Donna."

"Mom, I wish we would have kept our Barbie dolls; the first one was issued in 1951, and they would be worth a fortune now. My Tonka train is worth a lot of money now, too. Jeremy and I went to K-Mart and I bought a Joe Boxer comforter for less money than anywhere else — it has a zebra print on one side and is yellow on the other side. I love it, I love it! I will be able to turn it over in the spring and have it so sunny in my room. It was the only thing I bought for myself; everything I bought was for everybody else. I bought Hello Kitty PJs for Lisa at Sears, and she cracked up laughing when she saw them.

"Jeremy got the trail camera, camouflage green, sneakers, and clothes and lots of gift cards and money. Mom, I love making people happy and for once in several years, I've been able to give people presents without worrying about the cost! Even though when I got money gifts, I used all of it to buy Jeremy his presents. I am so blessed — it's been one of the best Christmases I've had in a long time! Thank you and Jerr for the wonderful gifts and money for us; you know we can always use them on something special — after Christmas when all the sales are on. That's the best time to shop!" ⚓ ⚓

While we were away from home for a couple of hours, Debra had retrieved our mail from the mailbox as requested. She found a solicitation letter from a St. Luke Children's Research Hospital with a photo of a six year old cancer patient. When we opened the letter, we saw the artwork and a poem of an eight old with neuroblastoma and he entitled it "B is for Believe." He wrote (sic):

Believe in your self because St. Jude is on your side. The fight may be tough But hold your head up with pride. It's going to be ok.

Live Life and Believe. It's OK to cry. It will be fine. We all have to believe they will find a cure one day.

Just remember we all have to Believe!

Debra sat with this letter in her lap and looked at the first little girl shown with cancer, then read the artwork and started sobbing. I hugged her, crying, too, and asked her if she was alright. When she could grab a breath, she said, "Gosh, Mom, and here I am complaining about my treatments and I kinda know what to expect — but how can they? How can they possibly know or understand what is being done to them? And why? How can God be so cruel to give these babies, little children or anybody this horrible disease? And with all the millions of dollars spent in research, and the brilliant minds and they can't find how to stop cancers?" (*In my opinion, I suspect the cure has been found but there's billions of money involved and thousands of jobs that wouldn't be there if a cure were found! Isn't that a irrational thought. I'm sorry. I'm upset. And one day someone will find this book and ask, "Cancer? What was that?"*)

2012

THE BEGINNING OF THE END

1/1/12, Sun. NEW YEAR'S DAY —

"Happy New Year, Mummy, to you and Jerr! Are you having your famous mimosas?"

"And to you and Jeremy and everybody else. Let's pray for a wonderful new year."

Debra again told us her new zebra comforter is SO comfortable, so cozy, and soft; she doesn't want to leave it. "THANK YOU again, Mummy. I love you both."

Personal: Jeremy is going to a tanning salon twice a month for three minutes to start getting tan for Florida; he doesn't want to stand out by being so pale and white. ⚓⚓ They give him a special sun screen with high SPF, special glasses and cream.

Lisa bought Deb PJ's, a red blanket, a plaque, and she had bought Lisa PJs, too. "Mom, we were both laughing — great minds think alike! Then I got other personal items — razors, toothpaste — things I can take to the hospital with me --- if I have to go again. You don't realize what you need until you go to reach for it, and you have a small little drawer that you can't reach and all your personal items are in a square pan. Do you remember when I got gifts like the beautiful clothes you gave me — jewelry, good earrings which you always split up between me and Donna because we could each wear only one? How I appreciated all the surprises, gift cards, and money, but these days, how much more I appreciate the little personal things now, too!"

1/3/12, Tues., 7:00 p.m. — Debra' call

She starts her first radiation treatment at CCS today, it took less than ten minutes, five minutes to register, three minutes to enter the treatment room, and two minutes for the radiation. "I love it, Mommy — no stress, no needles, no IVs, no undressing and such lovely people. Thank you, Mom. Why didn't I do this before? It was only when Dr. LaiLai threw me out of the room and my spirit was so devastated that I had the backbone to make a change. RPCI makes you feel powerless and under their control. Lisa drove me and it took longer to get up, get dressed, to drive there and back than it took me for my treatment! It was like going to the bathroom. Oops!" ⚓ ⚓

The doctor's office placed the request for van transportation for her; Debra didn't have to do anything — can you imagine? She didn't feel a thing, but she was tired and slept for five hours and just now woke up.

She and Lisa stopped at Dash's in our neighborhood and bought all the stuff so Debra could make her special, yummy spaghetti sauce! It was a little more expensive, but they were right there, and it was almost zero degrees outside. They drove the back routes home, and it didn't take them long. "I'm cooking again, Mom! You remember my sauce and the aroma throughout the house?! And at home, I was the microwave queen, I could play that microwave like a orchestra conductor — ding, ding, ding! Dinner's ready everybody!" ⚓ ⚓

1/3/12, Wed. —

Debra went for her radiation treatment. Medicaid has approved
her taxi ride to CCS. "The taxi they arranged will be picking me up
every day and taking me to the treatment center and back home."
She has to get a referral from her primary doctor, saw a social
worker who thought she had blood poisoning from Florida or New
York. She will see a representative from her insurance company
next week.

While Debra was in the waiting room for a few minutes, she saw a
water delivery man come in to CCS for treatment during his lunch
hour; another worker came in during her lunch hour. "Mom, it's
so convenient and people here are so respectful of a person's time.
All prescriptions are provided and they call into the pharmacy.
Once every week, I see the doctor to discuss my progress, and I get
a printed report every Friday. CCS has a robe with your name if
you want to wear it instead of the disposable gowns. The machine
looks like a huge satellite dish; it reminds me of a "Star Wars" set,
but in less time than you can blink, you're done; no taking your
shoes off; no taking clothes off, no **internal** exams with everyone
peering at your privates! There's a three-foot thick door which
looks like a bank vault, the machine itself is all open not like the
MRI. There's no pain, no feeling, you don't know anything is being
done to you. Amazing!"

1/5/11, Thurs., 4:00 p.m. —

Debra just got up, was a little tired, but didn't even sleep. She woke
up this morning with red cheeks and asked Lisa do you think this
is from the radiation? When she got to CCS, she asked about this,
and the technician asked if she had had chemo recently (Yes!).
She was informed that it takes months for that poison to leave
your body, it was still from the chemo. Her stomach and chest are
hurting and so are her arms and legs. "Again, in the few minutes
I was in the waiting room, Mom, I met a lovely lady probably in

her 60's, today was her last treatment, she had cancer in her chest and all over, had thirty-two treatments and it was gone. I feel so confident, it's good to have energy, to feel good, to not feel sick, or wonder if a pain or ache is going to develop into something else and I have to go to the hospital — something I always dreaded! Her hair is beginning to grow again, can you imagine?! She and Jeremy are now comparing the length of their hair. "Mom, my hair is actually light brown and soft and silky. It's like a little cap — or like one of those that Jerr and the Jewish wear? (*Yarmulke*). Probably when I come to Florida, I won't need to wear my wig at all! All my cancer was in the upper chest, and he was giving me a vaginal exam every time — why? It was never explained to me. I probably have a Million Dollar vagina! Lisa said Dr. LaiLai would have eventually killed me. Remember when Dr. LaiLai said he would probably kill me before the cancer would? Well, he was giving me a message, wasn't he? But it was probably a blessing!" (*Deb's last chemo treatment was 10/20/11 and she was told on 11/17/11 that RPCI couldn't treat her any more.*)

Personal: "Mom, my special spaghetti sauce turned out so, so good; everybody loved it and couldn't get enough! The aroma throughout the house was wonderful! We have enough left over to pack five jars. Doug makes his own applesauce, spends hours peeling apples, and he packs his own peppers, too. You can imagine the aroma from those!"

1/9/12, Mon., 9:30 a.m. — ICU @ NFMMH

Lisa called that Debra has been in ICU since Saturday night! She's stable and knows her surroundings. "It's really odd, but Doug came downstairs during the middle of the night. Debra had just walked out of her room curled in pain with a severe stomach ache which had worsened during the night. She had trouble sleeping and breathing and was in the process of calling 911. She was curled up it hurt so badly. She had stopped taking her steroids which did help her to breathe and sometimes she had to take two. Chris is still listed on her Health Care Proxy because he's there in Niagara Falls and "Remember, Mom, we talked about it because you guys go back and forth to Florida." Debra had to name another person — so Lisa was listed so she can get information if necessary." Lisa told the nurse this morning she was Debra's sister. (*I told her I know, that HIPAA* stinks, I can't get any information because of "privacy schimacy — that's my daughter. I need to know!"*) "I agree with you, Lorraine, this Privacy Act is for the birds! Debra has no phone in the room, of course, and her cell phone is at home."

Lisa: "Lorraine, did Debra tell you that on Christmas Eve, when she wanted to go shopping by herself, that people had reported her erratic driving, and she was stopped by a State Trooper on her way home? (*No!*) When he learned of her condition, he followed her home so that she would be safe. She was driving my jeep, and I told her, "That's it, Debra — no more driving my car or any car. Next time we go with you!" *When I asked Debra about it later, she told me "But, Mom, I wanted everybody's presents to be a surprise this year! How could they have been if I took them with me? I had a ball shopping with everybody in mind!"*

Personal: Lisa told me, "Debra called Phil and told him again he has to work with us; he has to either meet us halfway or all the way to bring Jeremy here. No more pulling Debra in different directions. He's aware of her condition. Jeremy is so stressed when he gets here that sometimes he takes it out on Debra, and I had to stop him. — 'No, no, Jeremy, none of that here.' She does his laundry here which I didn't know about. I had to stop her from going to the tanning salon with him." (*NO!*)

Later, I called OCC and notified Dr. Yi's assistant, Mia, about Debra's hospitalization, and she asked in what hospital was she and that Dr. Yi will immediately call the doctors there. (*Dr. LaiLai had never asked or even offered to contact her doctors!*) She's had pain in her stomach, probably her ulcers, not from radiation. She is fighting it but has trouble breathing, her skin was clammy. She called 911, then left message on her father's machine. The nurse finally told me she was stable and was talking and was aware what she was saying. (*Thank, God.*)

1/10/12, Tues., 4:00 p.m. —

In S-3, Room 349, no answer.

11:00 p.m. —

I called the nurses station and was told Debra was comfortable and was sleeping. *"Please tell Debra her mother called."*

1/11/12, Wed. 11:00 a.m. —

After repeatedly calling Debra's room and had no answer, I called the nurses station on S-3 floor, Rhonna checked and found that Debra's ringer had been turned off!

"Mom, my stomach is killing me, the pain is so bad; I was curled up and crying, couldn't even talk. I couldn't call you, Mummy. I've had dozens of tests, upper gastro, lower gastro, MRI, CT scan, I had the hose inserted in my nose again, couldn't eat anything. I'm so hungry, but now I'm on a liquid diet. I haven't been given anything for pain yet and can't take the Lortab. Why do they insist on giving me that? My skin is so numb; it feels terrible to the touch.

"I had popsicles for breakfast — so yummy, really — and now the nurse brought in coffee. When have I ever had coffee, but it was good; I drank the whole cup. I will call you after dinner."

Personal: Debra gave me Donna's new cell phone number.

"Mom, I'm so sorry for my language but sometimes when the pain gets so unbearable, I get so mad at it (the pain) and it comes out in my words — sorry."

"Sweetheart, if it was me going through with what you've been going through, you'd hear a lot worse language. We love you." "Mom, I know,

I love you two, too." Jerr and I discussed the situation and we wanted to pack and return home.

Another call. "I'm feeling better, Mom, eating potato soup without the potatoes! The doctor didn't say anything but that he's thinking about my condition and that if he can't do anything about it, he might have to change my treatment. My moods go down in an instant. (crying ⚥) It's exhausting trying to act normal when I'm not. Everybody wants me to act normal, and I'm not normal. I'm a sick person, sick of Lisa trying to treat me like I'm normal and I'm not. She's trying to cure me and she can't. I don't see her being in the hospital for a cold. This is something that isn't cured like a cold. I know I'm not going to be better when I get out of here. She thinks I don't want to do it. With her, it's day after day — I hear statements like, 'I have to go to the gym — I have to walk around the track — I have to walk around the block.' That doesn't help when I can't even walk down the hallway. Lisa takes so many pills herself — for sinus, for stomach, for everything! When I tell her my hips are giving out, and she says, "Well, Debra, you have to walk. Grrrr on everybody!"

"Debra, let's talk about you not being able to walk. I'm concerned about that condition. What do the doctors say about that? That's a rapid change from when were home a few months ago. What's happening?" (I'm *frightened and I'm lost in this situation and for once I don't know what to do. I've managed huge projects and community events involving thousands of people, and I can't manage my sweet daughter's medical treatment!)*

"No, I'm still sick. My red blood cells were down so I had blood transfusions again. I'm really tired of this, Mummy, really tired. I'm sorry for my mood and for what I said about Lisa when she and Doug have been so wonderful to me, I love them, but when I'm sick, I get irritated and impatient." "*Debra, it's understandable.*" (*Later I researched her meds and read that they do cause mood changes.*)

9:00 p.m. @ NFMMH —

Spoke to Lina, her nurse, she said Debra's stable now; the bleeding has stopped (*What bleeding?*). The problem has not increased. An X-ray was done but didn't show anything. The doctors will have to schedule another test tomorrow. She stated she can't give me any more information because of the HIPAA! She will tell Debra I called.

10:50 p.m.

Debra has finally heard from Social Security! They sent her two large checks and a debit card into which SSA will add funds every month. She stated again that she wants to send/bring her larger checks to deposit and for me to hold on to it for one year. If she doesn't need to spend it, she will bring the money to us in Florida so we can open a joint account — she wants both of our names on the account. She cashed the other check, and she still has all the money. *(We talked about this before. Does she remember?")*

1/12/12, Thurs. @ NFMMH —

Debra will not be discharged. She developed a fever of 101° last night. The pain in her stomach is better. Doctor said everything is better. Finally, she's going to eat a turkey sandwich! She was so hungry

Personal: "Mom, Jeremy went to a gym with a couple friends, so he's working out. His pain in his back is better, he's had me rubbing it. He must have pulled a muscle lifting weights trying to keep up with his dad or friends, but it's finally working itself out. This is another time I need to be there for him. I could have taken him to my doctor; which I will do if he's not better when I get out."

1/13/12, Fri., 9:15 a.m. — @ NFMMH

No answer in her room.

10:21 a.m. —

Debra is feeling much better. "My fever has gone down, Mom, but my potassium is low; my nurse gave me liquid potassium, and it tastes so salty. There's a huge blizzard today, in the last four hours, 5" of snow has fallen and another 5-6" is predicted. I'm staying in here; I'm not going anywhere, and I wouldn't ask anybody to come pick me up. But it's a good thing I'm not driving any more because if the doctor tells me I can go home, I'd get in that car and leave!"
⚓⚓

1/17/12, Tues., 7:30 p.m. @ E/R NFMMH —

Debra has severe stomach pain. She talked to Dr. Yi's office, and he said she probably can't take the radical radiation so her treatment will be revised to a regular dosage, instead of ten-to-fifteen visits, she will probably have to have thirty or thirty-five. Debra told me she was OK with that — whatever it takes, she was going to do. She was drinking the liquid pain killer, like Novocain, which only works for a short while. In the hospital, she can get pain meds by IV. She was 158 lbs. this summer and now weighs 120, losing almost 38 lbs. "I'd rather be here when I feel like this, even if I don't like to be here. If there was a medicine/pill I could take at home, I'd be happy with that. My stomach was like a hump-back whale, expanding out and back, it was so weird. I never saw that before."

("She's even been using "holy dirt" on her stomach! ⚓ ⚓ *You remember, "holy dirt" comes from a healing shrine in New Mexico called Chimayo where thousands of miracles occur; her great aunt and cousins from California made a pilgrimage there last year, said prayers for Debra and scooped up envelopes of "holy dirt". Bus tours of pilgrims and the sick and handicapped arrive at the shrine daily. The testimonies and hundreds of canes, crutches, wheelchairs, baby cribs and messages are displayed in the shrine. Tia Connie has sent us "holy dirt" in the past and it healed our ailments, surgeries, and other conditions. Did it really work?*

*How does it work? We don't know, we have seen the miracles and just
believe it in faith and it worked!)*

1/20/12, Fri. —

Finally reached Debra on her cell phone; it had not worked due
to low charge. She didn't answer my comment that when I called
Lisa's phone, there was a message that it was disconnected.

She and Lisa had just gotten home from her radiation treatment
today at OCC. Dr. Yi asked her all about her hospitalization and
her feelings, then told her she was fine, everything was fine.

1/21/12, Sat. 10:30 a.m. —

Her father calls me in Florida! He said, "Don't hang up, don't
hang up! I don't know if you know or not, but Debra was told
she has Stage 4 terminal cancer! We told Jeremy, he gets very mad
especially at me, when she was with Roswell, before she went
to that new place. Lisa knows. My sister, Midgie, has had Stage
4 cancer two times, she's in remission now. Deb said she was
broken-hearted about her own situation, telling me, 'I know I did
some not-so-good things in the past, but I've been good now for
seventeen years. Jeremy was the one who changed me. I know I'm
not telling you just to be mean.' And besides, you didn't....and one
other thing, you, and um um......."

*"Never ever have I heard about Stage 4 anything, not from the hospital,
not from Debra, not from Lisa or anyone. And whatever was going on
with Debra, she is the one who wanted to tell Jeremy in her own way, in
the special way that she and Jeremy communicate. You and others have
taken that right away from her. No one else had any business telling him
anything yet. How horrible for him to be told something like this and
with no follow-up emotional counseling — or being able to speak with his
mother about it? That's horrible. And why are we so morbid when doctors
are telling her she is going to be OK?"*

"(snarling) Don't you think she didn't tell you because she knew you couldn't handle it. You are ..... you........." *I hung up.*

I tried reaching Debra — no answer.

1/21/12, Sat., 4:00 p.m. —

"Hi, Mom, I'm feeling better, the pain in my stomach is much better, almost gone! I have an IV in my arm; I have to have sodium chloride to keep from getting dehydrated, a nurse comes to the house every day and checks the needle and the band aid which gets all yucky. I have to do this for five hours a day and that way I won't have to go to the hospital." *(She has an IV at Lisa's house to keep her hydrated; she has to have it for 10 days? I've never heard of such a home treatment!)*

"Mom, I talked to Dr. Yi's assistant, Dr. Yap. You remember I said he is a tall, young Chinese doctor with a great smile. He said everything is good, but they are going to lower the dose and extend the treatments so instead of fifteen treatments they are going to give me thirty, but I can't take the radical radiation that they wanted initially. My electrolytes keep getting depleted. I still don't know what causes that. I mean I know because we talked about it, but I don't understand. The doctor said the chemo should almost be gone from my body and it would be good sailing now with their treatment."

Personal: Jerr told her he still had the little medallion from the craft cart at RPCI which says "Believe in Miracles" and she said she does, too, and hers says "Angels of God". "Mom, must be why angels are always around me!" Jerr and Debra agreed that one day soon, he will give it back to her and we'll have both of them framed. 🔼🔼

1/23/12, Mon., 7:00 p.m. —

I had called at 5:00 p.m. and Lisa answered the phone and said Debra would call me back, that the visiting nurse was there at their house, everything was OK.

When Debra returned my call, she said she had a very productive day. She went for her radiation treatment but couldn't get it because the computers were down. Then back to Niagara Falls to her primary doctor, meeting him for the first time to get a referral for the radiation. He was really nice, a large, white doctor (as opposed to all the foreign doctors that are here). It took three hours to see the primary doctor, and she was not feeling well, but she endured the lengthy time — pacing, walking, sitting. The primary doctor was so relieved that Debra had her own pain management doctor. The doctor said his boss would be so relieved to hear that because they are having difficulty getting pain medications approved. A prominent wall sign states, "You can't get pain medication without having a blood test first." Debra had seen a documentary about pain pill factories where even nurses were writing prescriptions, they got in a lot of trouble, too.

She's having a visiting nurse at home only because the sodium chloride for hydration requires a needle and the nurse has to check it. Once a month, she has to have a blood test at the doctor's office, but the nurse that comes can do it although most facilities want to do their own testing. Now she's so tired, all she wants to do is rest. "My CCS doctor said after ten more treatments, I'll have another PET scan." She just anxious to just get started on her treatment schedule.

1/24/12, Tues. —

Debra went for her radiation treatment at CCS, hasn't call us yet. Then when she did said that Dr. Yi prescribed liquid Dilaudid, every six hours for the pain in her stomach from the tumor; she can get a port stick in her arm because of the needles. She said "Whatever needs to be done, as long as the stuff keeps me out of hospital. I'm so grateful for it, no matter how inconvenient."

A muscle spasm is blocking her airway; perhaps some side effects? Pain is being controlled with Lortab and Dilaudid. They make her numb. She sips water or hot tea all day; no more sodium chloride by IV; they took it out; don't need to have a treatment. She feels bloated — like a hump-back whale or a full stomach yet she doesn't feel like eating.

"Mom, it's really windy, with eight mph winds — so strong and it snowed a bit."

1/25/12, Wed. —

She told the doctor everything about her symptoms, medications and feelings. He's giving her something for nausea and a muscle relaxer; it will have a calming effect. Her symptoms shouldn't be from the radiation treatment; her body could be nervous; the more treatments you have, the tumor will get smaller. "Mom, I feel like when I had chemotherapy, why? I remember the nurse telling me it would be months before the chemo would leave my body — why do they inject you with this poison when there are other options? Dr. Yap is so nice, a real cutey."

1/26/12, Thurs. —

Personal: Jerr's older brother, Sammy and his wife, Faye, had a horrible car accident on Delaware Avenue. Sammy hit a fire hydrant, a street light pole, five cars, two which had just been finished at a collision shop and one coming in! The dashboard crushed Faye's feet, and she was trapped until firemen could cut her out. They were taken to Erie County Medical Center (ECMC), the trauma hospital in Buffalo. Uninjured, Sammy was discharged the next day. Plans to admit him temporarily into an assisted care facility were scrapped; he would not cooperate! Faye had been his sole caretaker. He became very upset and was later taken back to ECMC, and eventually was put in the same room with Faye.

Unknown to all of us, they were to spend one year at that hospital! During that year, after the surgeon's follow-up visit, no other doctors came to see them, only a few nurses — one who made the decision to reduce Faye's pain meds! She had a vertical steel rod in her right leg and a rod through her ankles to hold that rod in place! On their anniversary, we walked into their room to find her sobbing and crying out in pain, no one would answer her call button. I got Faye's permission to go to the nurses desk! The next day her pain meds were restored. We visited them every week, taking fresh fruit, diabetic cookies or hard candy, anything! The food was inedible, scarcely adequate.

1/27/12, Fri. —

Debra had her treatment at OCC. The doctor explained that the side effects could be from the radiation; that's just the way it's going to be until she gets better. She's very tired. Lisa came in to her bedroom and gave her two pills. She has taken Debra's pills away from her because she told me that at times, Debra was confused about all the dosages and times they were to be taken and missed some or took some twice. Now Lisa is keeping track. "I want them back, Mom. I'm not a child!"

1/28/12, Sat., 4:30 p.m. —

"Mummy, guess where I've been this afternoon. I've been out shopping! With the Munchkin, Jeremy. He bought sneakers, then went tanning, I looked at shoes and bought not one purse but two that I can take with me on the airplane to Florida and they won't charge me for a carryon — one leopard one and one in brown leather! They are so beautiful, I was so excited to find them; Jeremy had no idea how excited I was. I feel so good; all the meds are kicking in, and they are working. I have all the confidence in the world about this new clinic. Again, one thing they did was give me back my humanity. What a gift!"

1/30/12, Mon., 9:00 p.m. —

I've been trying to reach Debra all day. Finally, "Mom, I'm OK. I just woke up and thought it was 7:00 a.m.!" She had her treatment and has been sleeping all day, she's so tired. Her legs feel a little weak; she can't bend down. "The doctor really doesn't want me to go slow, Mom. I've been in bed for two years!

It's cold but not bitter cold outside. "

2/1/12, Wed. —

She has stomach pain, she's very tired; the pain doesn't go away; she's very cold, her legs are so tired; she can't walk.

"Debra, we're coming back to New York. I have to see you and hold you again. I have to make sure you're getting your treatments and meds and are being treated properly. I have so many questions. I want to talk to your doctors."

"Mom, I'm being treated. I'm OK, really. I love CCS and the doctors; they are so super to me. Can you imagine a doctor that actually sits and talks to you and listens? I know now that I am being treated better — for the first time in three years. Why did I wait so long? Everything will be OK. Please don't come back; you have to be in Florida and be there when I come with Jeremy on spring break! ⏏ ⏏

2/3/12, Fri. —

I called Lisa when Debra didn't answer her phone for phone for two days. She said she took it to charge as it was out of battery again.

Debra was sleeping. Her white count was elevated. Then last time she was in the hospital, she had a high glucose count of 239 and they want it regulated. Then later, it was still high at 159. She was asked if there was diabetes in the family. (*Diabetes? No, no one has diabetes in our family that I am aware of. Her stepfather and step grandmother had diabetes but it's out of her blood line.*) Her primary doctor is going to be told about the diabetes. She's going to have side effects until all the chemo is gone from her body. Also, Dr. Yi said her body is changing from the assault from chemo until now that it's getting better. There are no side effects from radiation. Lisa went into the consultation room with Debra.

2/4/12, Sat., 4:30 —

"Mummy, guess where we've been? (*She told me again about her shopping trip with Jeremy.*) I am really excited about two purses I bought; they are so beautiful, I am so excited to find them; Jeremy had no idea how excited I really was! I feel so good; all the meds are kicking in and working; I found Jeremy a "palm tree" luggage tag for his suitcase; he loves it, and of course, mine is a "Hello, Kitty" one! I was looking at the photos that we took on your patio this summer. I had always thought that wig looked good, but now I hate it — I hate that photo! I don't want to hear a wig to Florida, and I may not have to 'cause my hair is growing in so fast! How awful I looked in April; I'm not wearing a wig ever again! When I go to Jeremy's graduation, my hair should all be grown in. He'll love that. What a demoralizing experience for a woman to lose her hair! And why? Why? I think when you stop being treated like a human being and a woman, it makes your condition worse." (*The same would apply to a man.*)

She feels good; all meds are kicking in; has all tests done. "Mom, Jeremy keeps asking me questions. And I tell him, 'Don't I seem better, Jeremy? I've fulfilled my promises to you — you got your ears pierced, we went to Florida as promised and we're going again. We're going to Colorado (*hopefully*) to see a built-in theater in the Rocky Mountains — a River Rock resort that I saw on the Discovery channel. Mom, when he's 21, let's take him to Las Vegas. Will Jerr agree to that?" "*Of course, he'd love to go to Las Vegas. It will be a great trip — with a stop in Colorado? We'll see how that can be arranged, but it's no problem. Whatever you want, sweetheart, because that's what Jerr said he was wanted to do.*"

Jeremy's concerned about getting his hair gel expensive ($14) on the plane. I told her someone can mail those items like that on Monday, and they will be in Florida before they arrive. *(Please, God, let it be so.)*

"OK, I can do that no problem. Mom, I have money in my debit account! Yeeeaaah, as you would say! After years of zero money, nothing at all, and at my age, depending on you guys for my survival, it feels so good, really good that I can relax and take care of my finances. It feels so good to be able to buy items and not pass them by because I'm broke or not want to impose on anybody. You have no idea how demoralizing it is to be dependant on others when I've been so independent all my life! Also it feels so good to be able to eat without having a stomach ache."

2/5/12, Sun. —

I called Debra again; no answer; called Lisa and left a message. Now I'm really concerned again! Jerr and I have discussed closing up the condo and making arrangements to drive back home. We're going back to New York.

2/6/12, Mon. —

"Mom, I had a real good talk with Dr. Yi today. He told me my body is changing from the assault of chemo until now it's getting better. No side effects from radiation.". I told him, 'Dr. Yi, I'm resigned to coming here for 6-7 months. It won't bother me, truly. I've been going through this for three years. Just getting into this mode, I have trouble breathing but it's nothing to do with radiation. I keep having panic attacks. I'm not due for another PET scan.' I told Dr. Yi about my wonderful shopping day with Jeremy. He was smiling. It made me feel so good. He definitely thinks she's getting better than when she first went there. "I am definitely better, Mom. I met an Italian woman, elegantly groomed who told me that RPCI almost killed her. She was so happy she had gone to OCC. I agreed with her."

(Although, I was a candidate for the condo board and the election was on February 14, Jerr and I began packing to leave Florida. I felt such an urgency. Other of my obligations in the building and the City were inconsequential right now. Friends took up the reins for me!)

2/7/12, Tues. —

Where is my daughter? No answer on phone.

2/8/12, Wed. @ MSMH — Chris' call

Debra wants me to call her at the hospital; he gave me her phone number. She didn't take her cell phone with her again. After she talked to me on Monday, she went into the hospital with severe pain in her stomach, really, really bad. Tests ordered for her were an X-ray, a CT scan, and today a sonogram on her gallbladder. It was suspected her bowel blockage is back and not being dissolved with the tube in her nose and down her throat. On Monday, she had so much pain, she was delirious and crying; she didn't even get dressed; she went to the hospital in her PJs and slippers. Chris told us wait until you talk to Deb before you think about traveling up north.

"Mom, I know what gallbladder is but how would I have it?" (*I researched the Internet and read her the symptoms for gallbladder, and she had all of them.*) The surgeon will talk to her later today after they get the test results; she may have to have her gall bladder removed. She had to fight to get Dilaudid again, that she's been on it for three years, and it will not make her 'bounce around the room'! The nurses keep watching her, and she's fine, just not in pain; they are amazed. Day after tomorrow, Debra will have a colonoscopy… if the sonogram results are negative.

Personal: Debra asked, "Do you remember Cathy? She's a nurse at MSMH and her niece works on the 6th Floor and was stunned to learn who I was when she saw my last name. It must be Tommy's daughter; she's real cute, with short, spiky hair."

2/9/12, Thurs. — @ MSMH —

Debra will have another test again in a few days. The gallbladder is not inflamed, but there's a tumor pushing against the gallbladder. She has been put on a liquid diet; her doctor didn't say anything about the colonoscopy. There is a large Indian lady (worst breath in the world) came into my room wearing a winter coat and told her 'no blockage, not inflamed'. However, Debra was given another gallbladder test.

"Mom, if I'm in this hospital, I can't go to my appointments at CCS. Please call them for me, Mom? I had an upper GI series, and I didn't even feel the camera. Dr. Yogi, a doctor in his late 70's, says there's some food blocking the picture, and said: 'I couldn't see the picture behind the stomach to see if the food was blocking the stomach. It's going to hurt because it's pushing.' I'm being given antibiotics and pain meds every three hours."

8:30 p.m. —

"Mom, I took Holy Communion yesterday; the spiritual advisor looked so cute; I haven't been to confession but I'm accepting everything they offer here. I figure if I didn't die after two years of taking chemotherapy, I have a chance now so I better be prepared!" She told me that Lee at OCC asked: "Is Debra going to be able to travel in April?" Doctor: We don't know right now; we have to wait it out. Don't worry."

"And that cute smile; it's so nice at OCC. Mom, I can hardly wait for you to meet my doctors and everybody here. Patty, the nurse, goes above and beyond. She made all the phone calls for me to the cab company, the pharmacy, everybody — what a relief. What a surprise and it cures the stress — the stress of needing to do things and not having the strength to do them, or giving up your freedom and having others do them for me. That's why I try to do things on my own, until I just can't."

"Debra, Holy Communion? I remember when you girls made your First Holy Communion. You prepared for it and finally the day was here. You looked like little princesses in your lacy, fluffy white dress and veil. The photos showed you so devout and solemn. Then fifteen years later, you dressed like punk rockers for a Halloween party, black leathers, studs, purple lipstick, and spiky hair styles!" ⚓ ⚓ *"Debra, do you realize what a blessing and special gift it is that you were taken to MSMH because of their spiritual care to patients?"* (Oh, Debra, may you return to your spiritual roots and be blessed for ever. You have no idea how moved I was that you had Holy Communion and had prayers from spiritual advisors. God bless you, sweetheart.)*

"I know, Mommy, but it was not your fault that we fell away from the church. I can't really even tell you why. During our eight years at Catholic school and the nuns — we toed the line because they were so strict. And we had to be good, otherwise they would call YOU, and we would get in double trouble again! But they would find the silliest things to call me on — Sister would measure the length of my uniform. I was growing so fast that you couldn't keep up with lowering my hems to the 'proper length', and I would always get in trouble like I was — oh, horrors — a 'floozy' trying to show my legs to the poor little Catholic boys who cared less about the girls at that point! Although every time they said my uniform was too short, I would look at the boys and they were oblivious!" We laughed at the memory. *"And later about church?"* "Well, again, I don't have an answer. The longer you go without church, the more difficult it is to go back. And no one in the church really is in contact with you or even knows who you are."

"No, they don't know you or where you are, but God does, sweetheart. And Debra, you know where the church is and you know Father can be called. Even if you had come to church with me or asked me to go with you, it would have been so easy to just sit down and talk this over with Father. Jesus has never forsaken you, Debra. He has always had you in His heart and you will never be lost to Him. Do you remember those pictures of Jesus standing on the other side of a door and we are on this side? The

door on His side does not have a knob. We are the ones who have to open the door to Him. Well, what's done is done and in the long run, does it matter if you ask forgiveness at any time? In our faith, we've always been told, it's never too late. In one instant, you will receive God's forgiveness. He never abandons us and sent his Son, Jesus, so that all may be saved. You just have to do what you can now and in the future."

"I promise, Mom, I promise. And I've been sorry about all the things I might have done or said as a kid and the things I didn't do for you, especially when you were going through all that trouble with dad, and you were all alone. You must have been so disappointed in me. I love you, Mummy."

"I love you, too, Debra, my sweetheart. But do you know what? I always felt that a mother's heart has many chambers filled with love and with different feelings for the people she loves. There's no size or limitation in those chambers. But the things that your children do that disappoint a mother can not even fill a thimble! And mothers are forever, you will never lose me, just as Jeremy will always have you. And God loves you even more than we do. God loves you because of who God is, not for what you did or didn't do. And I can repeat that and say God loves us because of who God is, not for what we did or didn't do."

"Mom, you always make me feel so good — just like all the stories you had for us as kids. And sometimes I'm sorry I even say I can't deal with your phone calls!" "Debra, we all feel that way at some time or another!"

"Mom, when I was reading all your seminar materials before I stuffed all those envelopes, I've tried to live my life like what you wanted." "Debra, all of our lives are different from others, and you lived your life your way. Remember we loved that song?" "Mom, do you remember some of those stories?"

"Well, I am happy that what I say makes you feel good about yourself, sweetheart. Let me see — yes, I do remember one story in particular. The one about the elderly Chinese woman and the two large pots, one which *was cracked while the other was perfect? She carried the two pots hanging on the end of a pole across her neck. As she walked back and forth from the stream, the perfect pot always delivered a full portion of water and was proud of its accomplishments. The cracked pot arrived only half full, and it was miserable and ashamed of its imperfection. After years of what it perceived to be bitter failure, one day by the stream, the pot that was cracked spoke to the woman. 'I am ashamed of myself because this crack in my side causes water to leak out all the way back to our house.' The old woman smiled and stroked the cracked pot, 'Did you notice that there are beautiful flowers on your side of the path, but not on the side of the perfect pot? That's because I have always known about your flaw, so I planted flower seeds on your side. Every day while we walked back from the stream, you watered the flowers. For two years, I have been able to pick these beautiful flowers for my table. With you being just the way you are, there would not be this beauty to grace my house!' Each of us has our own unique flaws. But it's the cracks and flaws we each have that make our lives so very interesting and rewarding. You've just got to take each person for what they are and look for the good in them."* "Yes, Mom, I remember that one. Thanks for always making me feel so good."

Personal: Jerr and I continue to pack and close up the condo and leave for Williamsville. We have targeted this coming weekend for our drive north. The roads along the six states from Florida to New York are fairly clear now although our friends say there's snow in the mountains and tunnels of West Virginia and Pennsylvania. I don't sleep.

Personal: "Mom, Jeremy is going to the Police Academy; he sometimes has a hot head and really likes doing things his way. He likes Chris because he has no temper and he is so even natured. One day, the three of us were driving in a rickety truck which Chris had borrowed to fix, the wires hanging down from the dashboard; our knees getting tangled in them, bolts on front seat, it was rocking around. Jeremy laughed." 🛅 🛅

2/10/12, Fri., 2:30 p.m. @ MSMH —

Another whole day of liquids; still giving her antibiotics. On Saturday, she will have another test, a scope down the throat.

"Mom, tonight is movie night on TV. Remember the movie 'Wait Until Dark' with Audrey Hepburn, it's on TMC now. I loved it but it scared me; it was so suspenseful. Later, the movie that will be on is 'Meet Me in Las Vegas'. I've seen it before, but I love seeing it again. It was so neat to see the marquees where you took pictures of me and Donna every time we went, do you remember? We had to choose the same marquee for our pose. It was as if nothing had changed in all these years, but I saw us growing up year after year. It's just like the Disneyland photos you took over the years, and we had to stand by Mickey Mouse's floral garden at the entrance! Now watching movies is the big thrill of my night, can you imagine? I'm going to be here until at least Monday. I bought white jeans size 5/6, waist 28 - can you believe that, after all these years! The nurse here was talking about going to Ft. Lauderdale in May but she couldn't find the specials on-line for flights. Mom, I told her to look at Spirit Airlines." (*NO! — Worse airline!*)

Spiritual Care was administered today.

7:30 p.m. —

No answer on Debra's phone. *Where are you, my daughter?*

8:30 p.m. —

Debra will have the scope test tomorrow. She feels the blockage has gone down, but she hasn't had a b/m, yet hasn't eaten anything since Monday. She can hardly wait until after the test so she can have something to eat. She keeps waiting all day for a food tray! Her IV keeps triggering off the machine and beeps; there's probably air in the line. Nurses tried several times to get it fixed. "OMG. I'm back to that again. Just like a water torture — drip, drip, and it seems that it becomes louder and louder the longer it goes on!"

2/11/12, Sat. 6:00 p.m. @ MSMH —

Didn't have her test today, probably not until Monday, she was told. "Doctors are still trying to get this "poop" thing down. I'm trying to sip broths and soups. I would like to get my radiation treatments done; I'm very concerned about them. It's been nine days. What happens to the cancer without treatment?"

Personal: "It's been snowing about a foot and a half in one day. The news reporter was standing behind Channel 7 TV; it's still snowing but will finally stop."

Personal: "Jeremy was so cute, he whispered 'Mom, Mom, come here. Look.' He had pulled down his pants about an inch around his waist, and he had a tan line! Wow, he's ready for Florida!" 🛁🛁

2/12/12, Sun., 5:00 p.m. @ MSMH —

"Mom, call me back later; I just got my big dinner — broth, yummy!"

Debra talked to Chris; he's taking her to the fabulous Salvatore's Italian Gardens in Williamsville — the new restaurant now is Russell's Steaks And More — and then they will drive over to Salvatore's and walk around and see all the statuary and figurines and vast collection of the owner's father. It's a landmark, but Chris has never been there. We talked about the Whitney Houston movie we watched together; about the movies, about the Grammy's.

2/13/12, Mon., 6:40 p.m. @ MSMH —

No answer.

7:30 p.m. —

The abdomen scan was done today; scope test scheduled for tomorrow. She was given a suppository and it worked somewhat. "But, Mom, I have such a pain; I think it may be from the bowel or it's almost time for a pain shot. I can't talk right now; I have to call the nurse."

Spiritual Care was administrated today.

2/14/12, Tues., 1:30 p.m. @ MSMH —

No answer.

3:30 p.m. —

Test not done yet. Lot of pain today; stomach hurts a lot. She told the doctor, he didn't say anything to her.

2/15/12, Wed., 11:00 a.m. @ MSMH —

No answer. Later, someone answered her phone "Miss Debra's room". The lady was doing rehab on her room mate and said Debra wasn't there, but didn't know where she was and suggested a call back in half an hour.

2:00 p.m. —

No answer.

2:45 p.m. —

"Mom, I'm being given a drip to control my own pain meds, and I can press the button when I need it. I was writhing and crying and curled in a ball. I get stressed out every time nurses come in to take a blood test and I think they aren't going to find a vein. I so desperately need the pain meds but am terrified about the IVs now. My stomach is not inflamed but irritated; I don't remember what I was told. I think it was that the bowel mass has moved so it's going down yeeeah. Doctors ordered another abdominal scan. I keep burping the medicine I was given for the test. I asked the doctor, 'Can I drink something?' He said, "Oh yes, you can.""

8:00 p.m. —

"Mom, I'm going to get the hose down my nose and throat again to try to dislodge this lump. It had been ordered and I kept refusing it, because it's horrible and painful, but I need to have it done — this pain is horrible. I'm working with a gastro doctor. I will ask him how to avoid this bowel obstruction thing in the future." *"Do you have to take a stool softener, a laxative, or something?"*

"I don't know, Mom, but I'll find out and do it! Hospitals are so embarrassing for the patient, there are things done to you, and you have to do things and talk about things that you would never do before in public — it has always been so embarrassing."

2/16/12, Thurs. @ MSMH —

No information.

2/17/12, Fri., 5:00 p.m. @ MSMH —

Debra was given Spiritual Care today.

Ginny visited Debra today and is going to stay until Chris comes in. Debra went for an MRI contrast test this morning this time. She was out of her room for quite a while.

8:20 p.m. —

Debra had the tube inserted through her nose this afternoon. "It wasn't as bad this time, maybe because this nurse knew what she was doing. It's really helping to relieve the bloating and the pain. I was talking to the surgeon today, and she's going to give me two days on this tube and see how that goes in dissolving the blockage. The surgeon told me, 'I don't want to do surgery on you, Debra, but if you have a blockage, there's nothing else I can do but do the surgery' and Mom, that's what I'll have to do to get rid of this pain."

Debra had to hang up and call the nurse; she feels like she has to go to the bathroom, and it's a big deal since she has to be unhooked from everything and she sits on the toilet and hardly anything happens — call back in twenty minutes.

9:30 p.m. —

I spoke to the Charge Nurse, who couldn't give me any information, but she would ask Debra what she wanted us to know! I informed her we were packing to leave Florida for New York. Nurse: "If you're in a position to make that arrangement, I would." *(All this time, I believed that with treatment or with surgery that Debra would be OK and that she would complete her radiation and be cancer-free. I believed what she told us and what the doctors were saying to her. Now I'm terrified!)*

When the nurse called me back, she said Debra didn't want anybody to know anything about her condition, only what the doctors were telling her and she believes them. And she will tell others what she wants! "I'm sorry," she said, "but it's her decision." *(What's going on here?)*

Personal: "Mom, Lisa is with Colton in the hospital; he had to have his appendix out; he had the same symptoms as I did, but I knew my appendix was already out. Poor Colton and I feel so sorry for Lisa — she's had a lot to contend with."

(In between this, my friend, Linda, calls and tells me her friend Carol had the same thing, 10 days in the hospital, severe pain, bowel obstruction, caused by scar tissue from cervical cancer surgery, she wasn't not eating, had test after test. Thank, God. I hope so.)

9:00 p.m. — Ginny's call

Chris is very upset; she left her phone number and Chris' phone number, although she didn't think he could talk to me. Call!

9:30 p.m. —

When I returned Ginny's call, she was crying. "Chris doesn't think Debra is going to make it through the night (*WHAT*?!). She said there's old blood and the doctor said one week or one month; doctor said she didn't think she would make it through the night. If the tube does not work in breaking up the obstruction, doctors told her she could live a week or a month." (*I was ice cold and shaking.*) Debra was facing it. She asked, "Ginny, do you think there's a hereafter? Was it painful when your mother passed away?" Ginny told her that on the last day her mother just went into a semi-coma and then went to sleep.

Debra: Is there much pain?

Ginny: She was talking about dying, Lorraine!

Debra said: I want to go to Florida! I want to go with Jeremy! The floors here are a little cold. I'm freezing!

Ginny: My mom said the same thing; one breath she was passing away and with another breath, she was looking forward to more plans and more time.

"Chris said Debra doesn't want you to know all this (*Why*?!) because you'll fall apart and you have Jerry to look after. (*I had my daughter to look after, too!*) Her hands are very white; she's lost a lot of weight; but she's not morbid; she wasn't crying.

"Debbie wanted to talk to Chris as he's her proxy. She asked him, "Do you want your ring back, Chris?" "No, Debra!" The worst thing for me would be if someone calls you up and tells you. I — one hundred percent — think you should come home." (*We are!*)

Debra told Ginny and Chris what she wanted, "You can have everything of mine that's at your house." Chris asked his mother, "Do you think I should call her mother? But I can't talk to her; I'm too upset!" "Maybe Chris can tell you something that he heard at the hospital. He called me this afternoon; asked me if I could stop and see her."

10:00 p.m. — My call to Chris.

"Hi, Chris, what's going on?" Chris was crying, "The female surgeon said her bowel obstruction was bad; she talked to her about surgery, but there was no guarantee about the outcome. I had to leave the room, because they were going to do some exam and test on her. Her father came in with Jeremy about ten minutes before visiting hours were over. Debra had been waiting for them all afternoon. They showed up for a few minutes and then her father wanted to leave. He said,, "C'mon Jeremy." She doesn't look good; she wanted me to sit and talk. She said, "We have to face reality." The nurses came in, then we were talking some more. Debra wants the china cabinet from her apartment go to Jeremy. It meant a lot to her growing up. She took a few things to Lisa's in her vehicle, but she was cold, and she didn't want to finish. Then an hour later, she called from hospital and told me to call you; that if something happens, you decide what to do with her stuff. Those things are the family's stuff, I shouldn't have it and that you should know where it goes!" (*I'm trying to comfort Chris and I'm sick!*)

(*We finished our conversation in tears. I hung up and shaking and sobbing. Jerr had heard the conversations, and he couldn't calm me, he got a cold washcloth and pressed it on my forehead and just held me. I kept replaying the conversations over and over and said, "It's not true. Please, God, it's not true." This time I felt a silent coldness and that my prayers were not received.*)

After a long discussion with Jerr, we continued the final packing up the apartment for the season. The valet took our suitcases to the car. I had lists of numerous tasks to be done — but couldn't do them. I was in the bathroom throwing up and crying. Jerr was very upset and didn't know what he was doing either. He said, "Whatever has to be done, honey, let's do it." Our best friends were in and out of our apartment helping us with things. Repeatedly, they told us, "Don't drive — please don't drive. Ship your car and fly." Ship our car? Had never done that. How? Where? When?

11:00 p.m. — Debra's call

"What's wrong, Mummy? Your voice sounds funny." I told her, I was just a little stressed because we were leaving the next day. "Mom, what's the big urgency, the nurse doesn't know anything! The doctor said the x-rays look improved; she's going to give it another three days and watch for an improvement and then decide whether or not to do surgery. She also told me that I was really not a good candidate for the surgery so we will talk about it again.

.........."This room was grand central station today; everybody was here, what did somebody do — put out a bulletin to come see me? The clergy, Social Services, fifteen people — it gets on your nerves; I don't want to sit and dwell about it — like 'Oh, there's the poor little thing in the corner, pity her'!"

......."Oh, guess who came to see me? I hadn't really seen Ginny in two years. After Tom died, she couldn't even function. I told her, 'There's nothing you can do; but you get yourself sick if you dwell on it.' Chris has all this other family stuff to deal with; I don't want to add to his problems. We've been communicating a lot.

......."Me and Phil have been talking since forever. I don't want to get in trouble with Buffy. Frankly, I don't really care what she says, but this has nothing to do with her at this point. She will have to live with it. She can't change that Phil is Jeremy's father and I'm his mother. That will be forever.

....."Mom, promise that you won't let Buffy treat Jeremy badly. He doesn't need that — ever! I won't have it and if I have to get it straightened out again, I will. I can talk to Phil about it. Jeremy didn't ask to be in their situation, and he didn't ask for my situation.

He needs somebody he can count on and somebody he can talk to about stuff.

......"Now my father, he's an idiot, I'm sorry, Mom. He doesn't want to go out so Jeremy stays home and goes on-line. He can't listen to his music. Dad has been going nuts lately, as usual. He's another one, he comes to see me, 'Oh, Deb, blah blah' (whinny voice). Did I tell you I had to throw him out of my room the other day, Security handled it. He was bringing up all kinds of stuff from the past, over and over again - abut you, about me, about Donna.. He doesn't see the good stuff. I told him, "Why are you trying to hurt me, you've hurt me in the past, and you see how much in pain I am, and you are still trying to hurt me! Why?

....."I had to throw him out of my apartment in the past, now from my hospital room? Security was escorting him out and he yelled out in the hallway 'I love you, Debra.' No, he doesn't. The horrible look on his face, sneering, anger. Oh God, I don't know what to do!

"One day, dad told me, "I'm going to get you a car, Debra." "Really?" I told him. Well, I've been waiting since 1991, remember the Firebird when you took me to the dealer, we spent hours there, I picked out a car then went into Augie's office, got a good deal, I signed the papers then all of a sudden, nothing. You said you didn't want to do it!

"He doesn't remember being thrown out of Avanti's (*where she worked*). Any other person would have lost their job the way he came storming in there. He has to bring up old stuff; it gets me so upset. I don't need that, Mummy! One minute threats and the next minute doom and gloom; then all the mumbling. Jeremy tells me when things are wrong at dad's house. I've threatened dad that if I have to, he'll only have supervised visits with Jeremy, and I tell him, 'You better stop talking money with Jeremy; he doesn't understand that you'll never come through; all you do is use it to manipulate people.' Dad has no one else to talk to; he's a weirdo, and he's been acting freaky the last four days. I asked Jeremy "How is he at home"? Jeremy said 'He's weird, but I spend most of the time in my bedroom.'

"Jeremy has taught himself how to digitally mix sounds, it sounds really cool. He's becoming a recognized DJ. He goes to the gym. Dad was pissed that I gave him the money to go to the gym; such a big problem about nothing. Dad is so pale, he's lost so much weight; supposedly takes good (legal) medicine now for something, but he told me his liver is all wrong. No, then he told me it was the kidney that was bad. He has different doctors than the ones in the past yet he's still got the same problems. And here I am fighting to get better, and he has to slam me worst than all the pain here! I told Lisa, 'I can't understand how you could be friends with my father all these years.' Originally, they were the ones who were friends, my dad and Lisa, her husband, Doug, and her family. And then I met Lisa and I really loved her.' "I love you, Mummy and that big guy, Jerr, I love him, too. He always makes me feel better and makes me laugh."

Personal: Donna is back at her father's house.

2/18/12, Sat. —

The valet packed our car trunk; I found an old trip tik — Jerr said the roads haven't changed, just the information about weather and construction. Friends of ours didn't like the weather reports especially going through the mountains and tunnels of West Virginia. We said, "If we have to stop, we will."

2/18/12, 4:30 p.m. —

Lisa called: "We had a hell of a week. Doug and I visited Debra today; she's good at a fight and has been fighting her condition all along. She doesn't want you to come! There is stuff draining from her colon and rectum; she has a feeding tube and is on a pain pump. I went and talked to the nurse; the surgeon herself is harsh and doesn't have a good bedside manner. She said she's not doing the surgery and wants to start Debra on radiation!

"Deb always likes to do things on her own (like her room or her laundry), not a lot, but enough. Athena (*their dog*) whimpers when she knows Deb is sick. A couple of times during the night, Athena comes up to my bed crying and runs up/down the stairs until I see if Deb is alright. Right now as it stands, she's being taken care of — really.

"She told me, 'Debbie cried — what if I don't make it until Jeremy graduates — what will he do?' Up to now, she was still not accepting it. She knew she was at Stage 4 terminal cancer, but wouldn't accept it. Dr. Yi told me that he told Debra, they were talking that her bowel was dead.

"Lorraine, I want to get wooden platforms close to the floor, Deb is very insecure in a standard bed, she wants to be close to the floor. The one I have has drawers. I told her father to stop being so cynical and morbid and to stay out of it. I'm the one asking the questions and when I get the answers, I'll tell you. She said Jeremy is really looking forward to the Florida trip, but he's beginning to lash out, has anger issues that he never had before. Personally, I would come home, Lorraine. It will give her strength. Her whole thing is to come back home to us and take meds. I did take away her meds especially the higher dosage pills and give them to her when prescribed. Before that she would take them for pain, and if the pain wasn't alleviated, she would take another one."

"Lisa, how long have you known about this and why weren't we told? Why did everybody keep this a secret and didn't they think her mother should be with her?" "We were doing what Debra wanted and now it's getting very critical. It's time to come home; she's going to need you." *"We are, Lisa. We are on our way!"*

2/18/12, Sat., 11:00 a.m. @ MSMH —

"Mummy, I'm feeling all right. I had a b/m yesterday; (now crying) why don't I get better; I'm afraid. I've been told they are going to make me comfortable and see if surgery is an option; they even told me I might not get better. Doctors are adding to pain meds, morphine, OxyContin. They did an abdominal scan, something is pushing on my gallbladder and my stomach, I haven't eaten in over a week yet I had a b/m yesterday, so the obstruction must be breaking up. Yeeeah! Mom, remember how excited you were with my b/m when I was little? 👍 👍 *"Yes, sweetheart. I remember everything."*

"Dr. Yi told the doctor here he can help me get rid of the tumor; he can shrink the tumor. I will see if surgery is an option, but I've been going to the bathroom. I told the doctor here what Dr. Yi said, but he said it's not only that — there are other problems. They are going to help me be comfortable; what does that mean? Comfortable? How? I don't know where I'm going to go when I leave here. A social worker was just in to see what they can do for pain. *"Sweetheart, you are coming home with Jerr and me!"* Jerr: *"Honest to God, Debra, I wish I could take it for you. I've lived my life, sweetheart. I mean it."*

"You wouldn't want this pain, Jerr, believe me. The doctor can shrink it to make me comfortable; the hospital doesn't really want me to be here; I feel like I'm being pushed out of here! Do not say anything to Jeremy, please. Phil told me (*again?*) he's coming to the hospital, and we are going to talk, really talk. *When?* He tells me he'll be there for me, but he isn't. He's said so many times he would come with Jeremy to see me and he doesn't. But this is one time he has to!

"I'm told I can't take it (the drip) home, but they can give me something similar. Pain patches don't work; Lortab doesn't work so something similar to the drip I'm receiving. They might have to give me morphine, but I've said I don't want it! Doctors said I can't have a controlled substance in a private home so I have to be given something else. I guess I can't drag this thing with me (*the IV pole*). ☏ ☏ We'll see in three days; I keep getting x-rays, and they keep changing their stories every day. I don't want to say anything; there is other stuff in the airway; the doctors don't know how fast it's reproducing. I'm getting nutrition through the tube. But, Mummy, I wish it would stop hurting. Why doesn't it?"

I had to break in to say "Debra, we are on our way home. We're leaving tomorrow morning at 6:00."

"WHY???!!! WHY???!!! It's so far! Not you, too!" (Getting real upset and crying hysterically.) ☏

(I made up a story that someone in Jerr's family was sick and that he didn't like the way that person sounded on the phone and that Jerr wants to be there to see for himself.) Oh, OK, Mummy, then are you coming to see me?" ☏ ☏ *"Yes, sweetheart, you will be our first stop, and we are staying there! I want to meet the great doctors you talk about and (yes, I wanted to meet the ones who weren't!).* She immediately calmed down and continued talking for over an hour. (*Was this the medication talking or was it really Debra? Did she know?*)

Personal: "Why doesn't Chris confide in me? I won't tell him, 'See I told you so there was problems with your kids.' " *"Debra, think about this. Chris probably feels you have enough on your plate without this added burden. It's not that he's ignoring you by not confiding in you."* "Mom, my problems are being taken care of as much as they can. Ginny was OK; she brought me PJ's and fluffy socks from Macy's. I can wear the socks but not the PJs — maybe when I get home."

As we were preparing to leave Florida, I re-entered the apartment to answer a call. It was Dr. Nikolaychook, the surgeon! She said: "I need to talk to you about Debra's condition. Debra has cancer all over the body, her bowels are all encased, the fatty tissue around the waist called mentum is all caked, the bowel is inside that and all the fluids we are putting through the nose tube are not touching the mass. I saw from the CT scan that surgery makes no sense. I consulted with Dr. Largo, the general surgeon. The prognosis is we don't know how long she has left. The bowel has not broken up; she could have less than six months while we try to find the solution. He said he talked to Debra about Hospice who will provide symptomatic relief; and she said, 'NO, NO, NO!' So we don't know how she can go home and be treated. Dr. Yi stated that he can treat the tumors to allow them to shrink, but now it doesn't look like it will break up. It's a serious problem, very advanced. I'm sorry to give you this news."

(I told her we WERE on our way, that we were packed and leaving. I also told her I hated Roswell and Dr. LaiLai. I feel he was experimenting with Debra; most of our contact was with his secretary, who gave us misinformation, miscommunication, or no information at all. When I talked to another doctor, he asked why after one year did we not seek a second opinion and why during all the time she was treated at RPCI did she not have a PET scan? We had no answers for that. We were like dummies just going along with what THE EXPERTS said!) I heard her making notes and she said, "I'm glad you are your way home, and we will wait for you." We hung up.

We were crying. I was shaking. I called my best friend, Terri, and she immediately came to our apartment. Our best friends surrounded us with love. We called other best friends, Jo-Ann and Bill, the board president, Bill came to our apartment (Jo-Ann was out). We told him what was happening and spoke for quite a while. He then said, "It's not my business, but you guys should not drive!" Terri and I were sitting on the love seat, and she was holding my hand, and we were both crying. She said "I told them that, Bill! I told them that."

Later, Sereda started researching plane reservations and reserved a flight the next day as no direct flights were available that day. She called a car transport company and made emergency arrangements to have our car shipped up north. All we had to do was give them our credit card numbers. The valet unpacked our car, and we started repacking suitcases to fly up north. Sereda gave us a shipping box to mail the rest of our things to Williamsville. We gave her a blank check to cover the postage, and she shipped our box the next day. Thank God for friends!

We called Lisa. "Lisa, no one ever told us about Stage 4! When did you know it and when was Debra told? We are returning to New York, we're leaving right now. I've talked to the doctor and are so upset. I can't think straight. But we're leaving."

4:00 p.m. —

In the midst of all this, Debra calls: "Hi, Mummy, did you talk to the doctor? Isn't she nice? What did she say?" 🔺 🔺 *I told her a little bit about what she said, but not the whole conversation, that surgery was not an option.*

Debra: "I had lemonade the other day, it was so good. I was so thirsty, I drank about 6-8 glasses and told the aide do you have to take that away? 🔺 🔺 Boy, I wish I could get my toe nails done; they are so long, it's so disgusting. That's the first thing I'm going to ask for when we get to Florida, is a pedicure. Can we go together?

"My nurse, Mary Jo, tries to be comforting but she's not; she has a look about her that I don't like. She asked, 'Did you tell your family; maybe you'd better get your family here; you've got to face the fact, you're not going to get better; they have to know!'

Debra: 'Oh, right, Mary Jo, they're all coming in from out of town so you better get some chairs in here; they're ALL coming. Whoopie.' Why is it her business to tell me this?!

"The ministry lady is real nice and they come every day. If I don't want to talk, she just sits and holds my hand. I've only had Holy

Communion. After all this time, isn't it funny that I'm here? I needed to be here in this hospital this time, don't you think?"

8:20 p.m. — Debra's call

She went to bathroom but is so out of breath. Also the movie channel was showing "The Bodyguard", I turned it on and we watched the movie together — Debra on her hospital TV and me here at home in Florida, not being able to sleep. "Mom, I'll always remember you singing all kinds of songs around the house, but most of all the one from this movie, "I Will Always Love You." "*And I'll always love you. Debra, I'll always love you.*"

Her temperature is 102°, but she says "I don't feel that hot; I am being given Tylenol. I can't get my breath, I can't walk, my legs are so weak, I can't take more than ten steps, I don't know if I'm going to be able to come to Florida, Mom. "*Sweetheart, can we take one day at a time? Let's just concentrate on your treatment and before you know it, we'll be there. The future will take care of itself and we will deal with it. (I had prayed for the miracle; it hadn't come. Why?)*

"Mom, I feel like I have a cold coming on. I've been throwing up; I took anti-nausea pills; don't want to go home yet. Mom, I just don't want to spoil Jeremy's trip to Florida on spring break. He's been counting on it all year, has saved money, we have made plans. The other day before I was admitted here, we walked the entire mall and back. He gave me his arm; I was holding on to him, and he was helping me; we both bought clothes for Florida. We were so excited." (Trying to encourage her and put her at ease.) "*Debra, if you feel you can travel, I'll order a wheelchair and someone will get you to the plane, but it has to be cleared by the doctor. And you know what — we were going to be back home in a couple of months, anyway. That is why I made the reservations for you two out of Niagara Falls instead of Buffalo, because the airport is only a couple of miles from Lisa's house instead of 20 miles away in Buffalo. But if you can't do it, well, guess what, sweetheart? That's life. We'll cancel the tickets and reschedule them for another time. No big deal. You have to do what you need to do and that's the only important issue here. What anyone else wants is not important, not me, not Jerr, and not Jeremy. There will always be disappointments in life, and we have to learn to deal with them, especially when we have no control over them.*

Chris called her but she couldn't talk to him because she told him, "I turned the wrong way and pulled a muscle. I want to watch another movie, Mummy; we'll talk later, OK?"

2/19/12, Sun. 9:15 p.m. —

"Mom, Chris just left; I called him again to read the Proxy. The doctors are using the methadone, but in between those doses, I need something for pain. I was told, 'You will still have the drip' but I don't! Mom, it was taken out! Now I'm in a panic! Now I'm having pains in my stomach and a sharp pain in my back. Why are they doing that to me?"

Personal: "Mom, Chris and I had a real nice talk and I told him what I wanted done with my things. He said, "Whatever you want, honey.""

5:30 p.m. — Debra's call

"Mom, guess who came to visit me! Aunt Midgie, Uncle Bill and their daughter! We had a great visit; she is so bitter about her brother. She told me how he almost ruined her life and the lives of her kids by interfering and manipulating. 'He tried ruining everybody's life, including mine.' She said, 'Aunt Connie's kids, too. She was saying that he had counseling as a kid (*For what?!*") 'Our dad was wrong to stop any treatments.' Aunt Midgie is very religious, Mom, very religious and before she left, she prayed over me and gave me a blessing. She said, 'God can change that tumor. I was told four times that I was dying and look, I recovered.' Midgie's hair is highlighted, real cute, haven't seen her since grandma's funeral twenty years ago. Aunt Midgie is just a saint on earth; she will make me grandma's special canola — if I can eat, she said, looking at all the hoses surrounding me, and we started thinking what can we fit in those tubes — not thin spaghetti, but maybe angel hair?! 🔼 🔼

"The doctor is trying to get me off all these pills; I haven't taken Lortab for thirty days; that's the worse thing to be on; they push these pills on you; Lortab is so addictive; it makes people murderers and causes them to exhibit strange behaviors. But what is one going to do in the hospital? Remember we read in the literature they gave me that a cancer patient cannot become addicted to the pain medications? Thank, God.

"Oh, my nurse, Merry; she's just wonderful, she bought a condo near you in Florida, she's going to be a snowbird until her son graduates from college; she is just so wonderful; looks a bit older and stern, she is very structured and to look at her, she looks like super bitch, but she is one of the nicest nurses ever I've been gifted with. She sits and holds my hand and talks. She told me they bought a condo at Tamarack; her son and wife were somewhere there in Florida, and she wanted to be close to them. Just to look at her; you know they were in love. To go through your whole life without friends, family is really sad. I've had the gift of both."

Much later Debra said, "Mummy, with everybody coming together does it mean there's going to be a funeral? (Crying) (*To myself OMG, I truly hope not!*) "I feel so bad for everybody because everybody is going to be sad, but you'll have to deal with it, Mom. What I don't want is hysterical sobbing in my face.

I said, "That's part of life, Debra, there are good parts and some not so good, and we can't control what happens. Everybody is going to have to deal with whatever happens in our life."

Later:

Debra: "It might not even be that long, Mummy, (*I simply went cold and clutched the phone tighter and prayed , what could I say, what could I say?)* " Mom, promise me you'll get on with your life and everyone else with their life. Jeremy is so great, he's very mature for his age, he does his own laundry, vacuums, does his school work, does entertainment, everything. I remember, Mom, when we complained about doing the chores, you said, 'They aren't chores, they are training to be a mother (or father)!

"I need you to be more in Jeremy's life. Phil has to understand that and so does Jeremy. When Phil comes to see me, he wants you guys there. I want peace of mind; that's what dad just doesn't understand; he can't believe how loyal these guys (my former friends) are to me. He doesn't know about my relationship with Chris, I love him, I love what he's done for me and for Jeremy, and dad doesn't know my relationship with Phil. Phil told me, 'Thank you for giving me such a great son; he's such a part of you and that's the best gift we shared.' "

"Debra, I remember reading that there was a man who survived 9/11 by reciting "The Lord's Prayer" while he and others were descending the stairs to the ground level, and in spite of the smoke and pouring water, he suddenly felt the wonder of God's peace and knew that Christ's love was all round them. He said, 'I know with a certainty that I will rise from this shell, like a child fresh and clean from a bath, and I will be wrapped in the warmth of His love and His forgiveness and His peace.' Can you cling to that, sweetheart, and believe because as much as we love you, Jesus loves you even more."

(I told her we would be there; we would be there as soon as we could. "Wait for us, sweetheart, we'll get everything straightened out!" We hung up. I was sobbing. I still didn't believe what was happening.

I still didn't understand how some doctors told us there was no sign of cancer and the other one that it had spread and closed the door on her face.

I was pacing the floor. Jerr said, "Forget everything, let's just go. She's our girl and she needs us.") Our Father......Our Father......nothing!

4:00 p.m.

Dr. Hash called us and said: " We need to talk to you about my talk with Debra. I had a long conversation with her. I told her what the surgeons said and that any treatment would not be of benefit for her. Her best option was Hospice. She needs to be thinking about it. We will disconnect all the IVs and lines and put her on oral pills or liquids. Should she develop a headache or nausea, we can help her with that. She's terrified of the nausea feeling and throwing up with the pills. When she is more comfortable and we find the formula that works for her, she'll be better. We've contacted Hospice House in Lockport as we feel that's the best one who can be with her 24/7 and allowing family to be with her, taking care of her, too. In my opinion, it is an excellent place.

"I did explain to her that the cancer is all over. It's in her chest, in her belly, and in her liver. *(What? What?)* Any radiation on the cancer will not be of any benefit. We can't insert a feeding tube with those conditions. We have to continue with care." Dr. Hash told me that he had told Debra, "Debra, if I look at your face, I can't believe you're sick." *(Yes, she is beautiful. She has that Mary Kay skin.)* 'But when we look at the reports and tests, you have a bad disease and the information doesn't match.' We'll keep increasing the meds on Debra; it's a little tough, but she will be more comfortable. She will slowly become less responsive and come to a point where the organs give out; she will pass away on her own. The body passing — when we start pain meds, some are much better, others just deteriorate. She may have three days or a month, we don't know. *(Are you telling me she is going to die, that she's dying?! I couldn't comprehend even now what I was being told. Words were like coming from a tunnel, like my head was wrapped with cotton!)*

"The G.I. doctor said "We don't want to put in any more IVs. We'll start her on methadone and in that case, she can't be on any IVs. We will give it by mouth or rectum. She will become unresponsive, but if you observe her, she will moan, her breathing will be heavier, that means she is in distress and the meds have to be given. Hospice would be the best place to be when we start the first dose of methadone and observe her very carefully. Regarding morphine, she said NO."

I told Dr. Hash about my feeling about RPCI and Dr. LaiLai. I could hear him writing down everything I said. He said , 'I'm really sorry about your experience.' He was telling us that Debra was dying!! She was dying, and there wasn't anything that could be done! There was nothing that medicine or doctors or hospitals could do. (God, WHERE WERE YOU!!) We informed Dr. Hash that we were on our way and would be home tomorrow. We could talk to him and any other doctor tomorrow and discuss with Debra the Hospice situation. He will wait for us, he said.

"*NO! NO! NO! PLEASE, GOD, NO!*" I screamed as I dropped the speaker phone back in the cradle. I was sobbing; I fell to my knees by the side of the bed. My husband, Jerr, had tears, too. He just stroked my hair. I couldn't believe what we had just been told by the doctor. Why? After all this time, why?

A million thoughts and memories raced through my head. The doctors had always said that everything was going fine, but "Let's have more treatments, more tests, more medications, more hospitalizations, but everything will be fine." Now I hated all of them. I was pounding my fists into the bedspread, saying how much I hated the doctors and the hospitals and the phony people connected with them. I said the three swear words I knew, surprising Jerr who had never heard such language from me. Jerr said, "Sweetheart, we can't let this destroy us. We have to be loving and strong like we've always been. We have to show Debbie our love like we've always done."

I thought what do we do? We have to leave Florida now! How do we get back to her this instant? How long will it take? How can I tell her? Who do we talk to — a multitude of questions? I wrapped my arms around my stomach, and I could feel my daughter, Debra. I could feel her as I did when I first held her in my arms. (*Oh my God, my little princess, my sweet girl, what can we do for you, what didn't we do for you!*)

5:30 p.m. — Debra calls

"Well, did you talk to the doctor, Mommy? Isn't he nice, really nice, I like him." We discussed some of the conversation. She said she feels better already; the IVs have been taken out and

she had her first dose of methadone. "Mom, when the doctor comes to see me, he wants you guys here. I want peace of mind."

9:30 p.m. —

Chris was just leaving her room when I called. I heard her tell him, "Bye, honey". She said she called him to come to read the Proxy again and in between the reading, told him again about all her things and what she wanted done with them.

"Debra, sweetheart, what do you think is going to happen? Please tell me."

"Nothing, Mom, I just want him to know what to do with my stuff in case I don't go back home to Chris' house and have to go somewhere else, and I don't want any of those things lost. They meant a lot to you and a lot to me. What if I can't ever go back home and have to stay with Lisa?

2/19/12, 3:30 a.m. to 7:30 a.m. - 4 HOURS — Debra's call!

Debra called us! She found a way to bypass the locked phone system and had the hospital operator put a collect call through to us. I put the speaker phone between me and Jerr. She was crying;

her voice was hoarse: "Mummy, my throat hurts so much." (*Did you call the nurse, sweetheart?*) "No." (*Well, call the nurse, or can I call her for you?*) "No," she said, "I'll do it but I didn't want to bother her again."

In the dim light of her room, a little old lady with beautiful white hair stood by her bed and asked Debra, "Can I do something for you, sweetheart?" She told the lady about her throat which hurt so much. The lady said, "Buzz for the nurse but I'll tell her what you need." I asked Debra who that was and she said she must be a volunteer. (*I thought: At 3:30 a.m.? How strange. I've never heard of that.*)

"Mom, don't hang up." Debra buzzed for the nurse who responded immediately, asking if she wanted ice chips. She didn't because they hurt her throat even more, and then the nurse said "I'll bring you a spray." She brought a cherry-flavored Cloresceptic and sprayed Debra's throat. She left the can on her table. Within five minutes, Debra had relief and told me, "Now why didn't I think of doing that, Mummy? I've got relief, whew!"

(*I was silently praying, thank you, God, for sending someone for my daughter when I couldn't be there! We're on our way. We're on our way!*)

Debra then began incessantly talking about whether or not it would be appropriate to call some of her old boyfriends, could I find them for her? "They were very special people in my life." (*Debra had three long-term relationships. When they broke up, I felt the situation was that they wanted a family and Debra didn't — until Jeremy. Then over the years, it was "children" that most touched her heart and soul.*)

"One person I don't expect you to find is that famous hockey player that called me everything he played in Buffalo with the Buffalo Sabres — remember? He used to call you Mum! (*Yes, he was from Canada, she met him at the hotel one evening after a game and one of your friends that owned a taxi company introduced you. All the girls were falling all over him, 'Oh, you are great, oh, you were so wonderful on the ice, you were....blah blah, giggle, giggle.' You weren't saying anything, and he moved to stand by you. This was during your 'blonde' phase. You teased him and asked him if he had hit his finger with a hammer because his nail was black — and he started laughing! You didn't know anything about hockey pucks or the game, but you were so quiet and natural that he started calling you, and you spoke for hours and hours. One evening he asked me if he could invite you to his hotel for a late dinner in the restaurant. You asked if you should go and I said to be careful, and you walked into a roomful of reporters and friends and people! He did walk you to your car though. Later, he did ask you to move to Montreal and room with friends of his friends, and you told him, 'What, and leave snowy Buffalo?!' He's probably still laughing with you!)*

"Phil never stopped caring for me, Mom; we talked a long time; he said he didn't care what Buffy said. Debra told Phil what she wanted to happen with Jeremy; she wants Chris in Jeremy's life and wanted me and Jerry in his life. 'You are so loving and have positive influences on him.' Phil was OK with that."

She then started talking about how she thought she was having fun for thirty years but that the last sixteen years were the really quality times and best times. It all had to do with Jeremy and getting her life in order.

She remembered all the trips we took around the country, she loved Glouster and said "I want to go back there and see all the beautifully painted houses, remember we took a boat trip to see them? Can we go with Jeremy and show him?" (*Of course, sweetheart, we'll go anywhere you want to go.*)

"Jerr, remember when Jeremy got his toe stuck in your treadmill and he was bleeding? Mom was so upset but you calmly took care of the situation. Jeremy remembers that day. Or when Jeremy wanted a quote from Jerr because he had to read two books — one called "Milkweed" — about a Jewish orphan during the Warsaw,

Poland takeover. Jerr, born in Cuba, gave Jeremy that Jewish phrase, what was it? "Arbeit macht frei" (*A German phrase meaning "labour makes (you) free."*)

"Mom, then the day Jeremy was getting off the bus in a blizzard at 3:30 p.m., and there was no one to pick him up. Phil called me that he was forty-five minutes away so Jeremy had to walk home, and he didn't have a key to the house! All these things have hurt me because I wasn't there to protect him, or care for him, or hug him and make him hot chocolate when he's cold, or give him cold drinks when he's hot and sweaty. But there have been other events that made me glad. Please protect him and take care of him.

"Mom and Jerr, you were always so special to Jeremy. Remember when you took him to Toronto to see "Lion King". He never forgot it! Or to "Lion Country Safari", or to special movies, to all the festivals and boat tours in Lockport to see the canal locks or to Canalfest in Tonawanda. You bought him a unique motorcycle telephone, you got us matching red Christmas sweaters, and anything we needed, you made it special. Please stay in his life; he needs your positive influence.

"Mom, remember Florida years ago — when you had taken me and Donna to one of your conferences at The Diplomat Hotel in Hollywood, and when you were robbed in one of the conference rooms and your purse with everything in it was gone? You said you were never, ever going to return to Florida, and years later you guys ended up buying a condo right across the street! ⚓ ⚓ And even in spite of the problems back then — with no credit cards, no money, no plane tickets (until your company took care of everything for us), you continued with our scheduled tour of southern Florida, the orange groves, the tower, Disney World, everything else that was beautiful about Florida. You gave us such great times and showed us places that we never knew existed.

"Do you remember Colorado and the mountains? I want Jeremy

to see where I was born and where you were born and went to school. Then you took me and Donna to Arizona to another one of your conferences, you rented a car and Donna and I drove all around the desert. Donna fell in love with the area and didn't she go back years later and moved and bought a house there? You were so sad about her being so far away.

"Do you remember the blizzard we drove in to Syracuse to a seminar you were doing. I was so scared but you just kept right on driving, very calmly? You've been honored with every award, you worked for one company for twenty-five years, you had your own public speaking company and took us to some of your seminars, we even helped with collating materials — I thought we'd never finish! ⚓ ⚓

"Donna and I were talking about you last week. Donna said people don't realize how amazing Mom was. She took care of us, worked for an International Vice President, was involved in the community and in government, was 2nd Runner-up for International Secretary of the Year in Vancouver, B.C. — from the whole world! Not even Jerry and their family or friends realize, I don't think. You started many community projects — huge ones. Remember when you even involved us in creating a display for the Festival of Lights of Niagara Falls which you helped start? You started the clean-up of the city and made us participate — but we were so proud of our section, and you let me plant the flowers. You took me to your meetings with the NYS Seaway Trail. I used to tell people that me and Donna were in Who's Who of American Women. They asked how? I would tell them we were born to a famous woman — our Mom! I remember other names from that book — Nancy Reagan and Cheryl Ladd. We always called you "Our Big Lady."

"Big Lady! Debra, I know! All your school friends called me "big lady" too, and they really didn't know why — only that you did. Remember when some of your friends ran away from home, and they ran away to our house! The father and brother of one boy finally came to our house, and

I told him, he's OK, just give him a couple of days. He said, "Whew, we were so worried. I wanted to call you but didn't want neighbors to know of our problems." I told them, they aren't problems, just teen adjustments. We all sat on the family room carpet in front of the fireplace with only the Christmas candles on and talked and talked. The next day, they wanted to go home. That's how you met Chris by the way." Yea, I know, Mom. Oh, man, I can just picture that beautiful family room, so warm and cozy. Everybody loved our wallpaper and colors. WOW.

"Later, I was so nervous when you went to Europe all by yourself to visit your lifelong friends. All kinds of thoughts went through my head, what if I lost you, what if something happens, and we don't hear from you again. I thought of never hearing your voice ever. Anyway, I just hugged you, said 'I love you, Mommy, have a great trip.' Then to hear that Brenda and Robin surprised you with a trip throughout many countries! You have no idea how relieved I was when you came home (before the days of cell phones!) Then you started flying to England twice or three times a year. You promised us a trip with you one of these days — will we still go, Mom?

"Remember when Brenda and Robin came to Niagara Falls? One night after dinner, Donna sped off with Robin in her sports convertible and we thought we'd never seem then again. I think Brenda was so relieved when they did finally return to the hotel. You were the greatest tour guide to everybody who came to Niagara Falls, Buffalo and Toronto — no matter what part of the world they were from. I would be amazed at the amount of knowledge you had. We had the chance to meet people from Russia, Egypt, Africa — people we never would have had a meal with and talked to across the table.

"And Jerry, when you and Mom went to Cuba as missionaries and later we sat for hours looking at your pictures and all the medicines you had to take. I was amazed that you had the courage to do that, knowing the situation there. Later, when you told us about

Communism and the dire poverty, I realized how lucky we were to be in America and to have all that we have. Jerry, will you take me the next time you go there? I want to see all those cool 1950's cars. (*You bet, my girly, girly.*)

"Jerry, take care of my Mom, you are the most wonderful person for her — the two of you together are such an example to me." "We *love you, Debra.*" Debra: " I love you two, too. Jerry take care of my Mom."

There was much more she was remembering. When she finally hung up, she said she was in such pain in her stomach that she just wanted to sleep. Then......

(*Little did I know that this would almost be the last time we talked to her — or heard her sweet voice. What we said to Debra was not as important as was her reminiscing about memories from years past. How strange that she would remember these long-ago situations and recall them to us at this time!*)

2/19/12, Sun. —

When we hung up after this four-hour conversation, I sat and cried and cried and was gasping for breath. Jerr was had tears, too, and he was just holding me in his warm, loving arms. Not able to sleep any more, we talked and cried and saw to the last things that needed to be done. How blessed we are with our friends, Terri and Sereda, then Sue came to our apartment with a note that she said "Don't open this for a couple of days, but you need to read it." She, too, had tears in her eyes. I didn't have an opportunity to read it for four days but when I did, Sue's beautiful suggestions to me about talking to Debra and stroking her face and hands were all things that we had done!

7:45 a.m. —

Our best friends in Williamsville, Lew had called us as we were preparing to leave for the airport and when I answered, he said "What are you doing there? You should be on the road already." I explained to him what was happening and how all our plans had changed and that we were now flying in. He asked "What time is your flight, I'm picking you up." We told him it was not necessary as we were renting a car. He said, "No you're not, Sandra is giving you her car!"

We were so anxious to get to the airport and in spite of the time, I wanted to get there early. I wanted the flight to leave on time, the plane to speed through the clouds so we could reach my daughter. Terri took us to Ft. Lauderdale Airport in spite of hectic business days during tax season and her overload of clients.

11:00 a.m. —

I called Debra and told her we were at the airport and coming home.

Debra: Will you be able to come see me, Mummy? (*Of course, sweetheart, I told you that you will be our first stop this afternoon. We love you, sweetheart."* She started crying, "Mummy, I am in so, so much pain, I can't stand it. They say I'm being given pain meds but it doesn't feel like it. I can hardly breathe because of the pain."

"Sweetheart, I'll be there; we'll be there with you; I want to hold you and hold you, just like I did when you were born; I couldn't put you down, you were so beautiful, and you are still so beautiful. I want to put my arms around you and sing in your ear and stroke your beautiful face.

Debra: "I love you, Mommy. I love you, Jerr. Thank you for being there for my Mom." He gasped for breath and told her, "I love you, sweetheart."

"We love you, too, Debra. We'll be there. We'll be there for you. We'll be there for you always!"

Debra: "I know, Mommy. You always were." (*Debra's final gift.*)

11:00 —

Donna told Debra that her cell phone kept breaking up and she had to go outside to call me back. Out in front of the hospital, Donna was sobbing and said Debra had been with her for her whole life. What was she going to do without her? We told her we were on our way. (*During the day, Debra kept saying we had called her from Pittsburgh and were on our way, and we would arrive in a couple of days.*) *Donna had been with Debra these last days. She had taken her sketch book, had helped her write a "bucket list", had cried, laughed, and held her. They were together always.*)

1:30 p.m. — Our Jet Blue flight, Ft. Lauderdale to Buffalo, NY couldn't fly fast enough. I was holding Jerr's hand and I was shaking — inside and outside. I was numb.

2/20/12, — Mon., 5:30 p.m. —

We arrived in Buffalo and called Debra's room; no answer.

Lew was at the airport to pick us up. We dropped our luggage at our condo at Hickory Hill, and Lew handed us the keys to Sandra's car, and we started out for MSMH in Lewiston. Donna called as we were at the Grand Island Bridge to tell us to exit the expressway at Witmer Road as the Lewiston-Queenston Bridge into Canada was severely backed up, and that we would never get off. Because of the holiday; the Canadians had been here in the area shopping for three days and were now returning home — there was a huge lineup on the expressway. When we got there, we took the Witmer exit, and when we were by the water towers on a road that parallels the expressway, we saw the lights of hundreds of cars and trucks in all lanes just standing in line!

About 7:20 p.m. —

We arrived at the hospital. Donna came out of Deb's room #624 and told us, "Debra was given pain meds this afternoon because she was in such distress and she hasn't woken up yet!"

When we walked in the room, I was shocked at my daughter's

appearance. Her head was turned toward Jeremy but she was unresponsive. Her eyes were closed and her breathing was erratic and gasping. Her arms were just lying on each side of her. Jeremy was sitting by her bedside holding her hand and crying and just looking at her. We went up to her and tried to hug her and kiss her and stroke her head. Donna, Jeremy, Chris, Jerr and I just hugged each other. We talked to Lisa and Doug who were there, I believe, but they left shortly thereafter. Everything was in a haze.

Her nurse, Kim, came in and said she had been there during the day, and the reason Debra was asleep was because she had been given methadone and another pain med. "The doctor has given her a 'muscle relaxer'. Chris had approved it." (*Why had the doctor ordered the "muscle relaxer" when he knew we were on the way? He knew we were coming back! Why? Why? Where is the doctor, may I speak to him? Why did he do that to her and to us? What was this? We have never been able to find out. Our requests for medical records have been not been responded to. Jerr said, "If she was in so much pain at eleven o'clock, sweetheart, would you have wanted her to lay there until we got here this many hours later? Whatever she was given at least made her comfortable, and we'll talk to her tomorrow." "OK, Jerr you're right, but, I'm staying right here!"*)

When we talked to Chris, he said he was with Debra at about 3:30 p.m. and that Deb had been given pain meds and 10 minutes later, she asked Chris to call for more, and he said, "Honey, it's only been 10 minutes." But went out and spoke to the nurse. She was then given a "muscle relaxer" to which she agreed because her body was tensed up because of the pain. Chris said he didn't really understand the whole story when he was informed and then agreed to the shot! He was devastated! Debra had drifted off to sleep and they couldn't awaken her!

The nurse informed us Debra was going to be given her Dilaudid tomorrow, and I said, "Good, that's the only pain med that really gives her comfort, not Lortab, not any of the other meds that the doctors have tried." (Later I thought, **now** they are willing to give her Dilaudid?! *I'll speak to the doctor tomorrow.*)

I asked her nurse, Kim, if Debra could hear us, and she said, "No, we will hear her moan or if she shifts in a way, we'll know she still has distress." She said normally it would be time to give her a pain shot of Dilaudid, but that they will discontinue them. I told her, "No! I want her to keep getting them. We don't know what she's feeling inside, I want her to continue to have the pain shots." We were talking quietly in the hallway. Kim said Debra should be more alert tomorrow morning and that Hospice had been there and that Hospice was returning tomorrow to talk to us at 1:00 p.m. (This was one of our earlier phone conversations Debra and I had. She said Hospice coming in without notice threw her in a panic, and she sent them away, saying. "Why was Hospice here? I didn't ask for them! Why were they going to take me away without ever discussing anything with me? Hospice wants we to go with them, they don't cover any care; they watch you lay there and die; don't even make sure you're eating! Donna wants me to go home with her. Jeremy gave me his room at dad's. I was cut off from insurance, in between if you're having a pain, they give you two pills of morphine, then again two hours later if it doesn't work and……..."

I remember one of our earlier conversations. *"Debra, why did Hospice come in there? Didn't they know we were on our way? I spoke to the doctor, he knew we were on our way!"* "My father and Lisa are scheming. I'm not a candidate for Hospice; what the hell is she doing here? I've been cut off from radiation; I'm mad! Stop b/s ing me I told them; it's not written in the report! I need Dilaudid and a drip, not the short-acting morphine pump; it gives me a headache. Honestly, Mom, I hope I go in my sleep or die from a heart attack! Donna is off next week; she's going to clean up Grandma's room. She's already changed, Mom and has been crying her eyes out and helping me so much. Without you, the reality now is that you were the strong one! All the games dad's played with Donna and now with Jeremy. I bite my tongue; I'm dying right now — big deal, they will give me something in five minutes — liquid morphine......

"I woke up today and comforted I'm not, Mom! I'm not going to be resuscitated! I am not living on a machine; nobody knows what I want to do! Fifty people coming in here for a week and a half and no one asks my opinion or what I want! I have no hopes; the hose is not draining my stomach; the machines have been turned off! I'm not going anywhere! I want to go home! They want to get rid of me here, well, send me home! I want to go home!"

"Debra, we'll be there and we'll deal with it. We will take you anywhere you want to go, and we'll deal with the doctors and the hospital. We'll all talk and decide what to do and make sure you're comfortable with your decision."

Donna had brought Deb her sketching pencils and pad (both Debra and Donna are artists). Donna had written a note for Debra in case she woke up before she returned. Earlier this morning, Donna had called to ask us if she could pick us up at the airport. I told her about our conversation and the offer by Lew and Sandra. Donna then told me she was in "Horn's" room (*her nickname for her sister*) that morning and that Debra said she was writing her "memoirs" and that a movie was going to be made of it! I had heard Debra chuckle with Donna. 🔱🔱 Mom, we wrote a "Bucket List" and it was all about Jeremy. (*Bucket List!?*)

When we walked into Debra's room, I was shocked. Our little girl's eyes were closed, her arms were on her sides and she didn't wake up when we spoke to her. We hugged Jeremy and repeated to him what the nurse had said, then when he stood up and came to the doorway, I told him *"This really sucks, doesn't it, Jeremy? You were her whole life, she loves you very much, but we don't want her to be in pain either."* He said, "I know, grandma. I'll be back tomorrow morning."

His grandfather was there when we arrived; he was leaning against the wall in the hallway, and I truly didn't recognize him after thirty-nine years! He looked so unkept, just like a little old man. He was muttering to himself, or to Doug who, I believe, was standing next to him. I couldn't even think, After a few minutes, the four of them left.

Chris went back downstairs and helped Jerr find the light switch on Sandra's car because we couldn't turn the headlights off! We were with Debra. I tried to hug her and put my arms around her. I was holding her hand and talking to her and told her, *"We're here, sweetheart"* and how much we loved her and how beautiful she was to us. She never moved or stopped her erratic breathing. The nurses introduced themselves to me and said they had been with Debra all day. (Donna later said, "Not true, Mom. No one came to her room — not while I was here!")

About midnight, 12:30 a.m. The nurse quietly told us, "Debra will sleep and you should go home and get some rest." I asked her, "Are you sure she won't wake up; she was waiting for us. Can you call us and we'll come right back?" She said, "We don't know, but she's resting, and yes, we will call you." Around 2:30 a.m., we left the hospital.

(Here I want to say that earlier when we arrived at the hospital, I asked the nurses who the little old lady volunteer was at 3:30 in the morning, that I wanted to thank her for her calm, loving words to Debra when she was in such pain. I was told "What volunteer? There are no volunteers at 3:30 a.m. and no one that answers that description!"OMG!)

Seeing Tim Horton's open and people inside, *(REALLY! We couldn't believe it.)* we stopped and had hot chocolate; got home about 3:30 a.m.

2/21/12, Tues., 3:30 a.m. —

I called the nurse's station and spoke to Vicki who called Bridget, Debra's nurse. She said there was no change in Debra's condition.

She was still groggy and has not woken up and had run a little temperature, 99°, and she was given a suppository. Again, I asked that we be called if she did wake up and to please tell her we are here.

8:30 a.m. —

We returned to the hospital, there was no change in Debra's condition. Her eyes were still closed; she hadn't changed her position. Her hands were still on each side of her body, she was now gasping for breath. The nurse came in with a handful of syringes and told us, "We're discontinuing her pain meds." I said, "No, you're not! I want Debra to continue having them. We don't know what is going on inside her and what she is feeling or not feeling, but I want her to have her pain meds." She said, "You want to continue her Dilaudid?" I said, "Yes, please." Then every six hours, a nurse came in and gave Debra the Dilaudid. Was it really Dilaudid? I don't know. All I know is that it was same looking syringe and labels that we had seen before.

11:30 a.m. —

I called, my sister, Chickie, and told her about Debra.

Right after noon, maybe 12:30 p.m. —

Lisa came to the hospital, said she wanted to speak to me privately. We didn't know where to go, so we stepped into Debra's bathroom and closed the door! She handed me an large envelope containing Debra's checks and cash money and said it needed to be deposited immediately — today! Lisa said, "You need to find your bank branch. Debra wanted this money put aside for Jeremy and to tell him 'Your Mom left this for you, for your college.' She said, "You can't ever tell Jeremy what we did." (*In the long run, what difference does it make now? Lisa eventually did tell Jeremy herself!*)

I put the huge bundle in my pocket under my suit jacket, and when we came out, I whispered to Jerr, "Come on, let's go find you someplace decent to eat instead of the hospital cafeteria." He looked at me ready to say no, that we had agreed to treat every-body downstairs, but I tugged on his arm. We made an excuse to Donna and Jeremy that we would find a café somewhere. (*This was certainly not like us because Jerr invites everybody anywhere for any meal — he includes everybody!*)

We left to find our bank branch. After stops at two other banks, one cashier told us their ATM wasn't working to go to their other branch in downtown Niagara Falls (*No.*). Finally, finding our bank branch, we deposited Debra's money and checks — all the money she had been saving for Jeremy.

Earlier, we had asked Donna if their best friend, Jason, could come to the hospital with his guitar and sing to Debra. The three of them had known each other forever growing up. Unfortunately, while Jerr and I were out finding a bank, he came to the hospital! He sang to Debra. Donna recorded "Amazing Grace." We were so sorry we had missed him, but he will sing at the funeral. Jeremy said he could arrange for the recording to be entered into a com-puter and hooked up to the system at the funeral home.

Later that afternoon, I was holding Debra's hand, and began singing to her "Jesus loves you, Jesus loves you." — then the rest of the verses. (*Jeremy stared at me; he probably didn't know that I could sing and probably never knew of all my performances here and in Canada.*)

When we returned to the hospital, Donna's father was out in the hall talking to Doug and gritting his teeth and sneering at me. He kept saying he had been to the funeral home (*funeral home? OMG!*) and had made all the arrangements and that I needed to give him $15,000 and he wanted a check now! Then he came into Debra's room and kept agitating me. This was Jerr's first view of my former husband! Jerr and I looked at each other and just kept quiet.

He kept carrying on this discussion as both of us were sitting across from each other at the side of Debra's bed, and he was still making statements about the funeral and the money and that I'd better give it to him now! I whispered again, *"This is **not** the time to discuss this and especially not here!"* He said "The hell it isn't, I want the money!" I told him, *"You are not going to have this discussion while my daughter is still breathing."* "Oh, your daughter, your daughter, huh?" Then he would mumble, mumble and lean over and put crosses on Debra's forehead.

That evening, Chickie and her two daughters, Janet and Amy, came in and spent over one hour with us. Chris and Ginny were also there. It was a wonderful evening under the circumstances.

Amy: "I didn't know who Tim was, I thought that he was with someone else; he looks like a hobo, really creepy." As a medical professional, she said he looks mental. Amy doesn't really have bad memories of him; she was too small when all the divorce stuff was happening, and Donna and I had to seek sanctuary at Chickie and Steve's house. When Amy finally recognized him, he whispered "I know who you are, you're my goddaughter." Amy said, "No, I'm not, that is Janet." Amy sat with Debra for a while, and then when Janet came in, talked to Debra and Janet sat on the side of the bed holding her hand. All of us were quietly talking and sharing stories about the pranks the four cousins had pulled and the other secrets they had, and we were quietly giggling about all the episodes. (*Now I'm finding out about these?!*) Later, Janet said Debra pressed her hand!! OMG Also, later, Chickie said Steve told her, "I hope Lorraine doesn't mind, I don't know how'll how he'll react when he goes to the funeral home, but he hated Tim with a passion for what he did to our families!"

When everyone left and the five of us remained with Debra, her father who wouldn't leave, kept up the comments, the threats, saying he wanted the money now. By this time he had moved to the chair at the foot of Debra's bed and next to Jerr. I saw Jerr fisting his hands, so I stood up from the side of Deb's bed and just tapped Jerr's hand lightly and walked over their legs. Tim said

"Where do you think you're going?!" *"I'm going to call the nurse. My daughter doesn't need to hear this from you."* "Your daughter, s***, your daughter." *"Yes, Tim, she is MY daughter."* "Oh, yes, the nurse! You think I'm scared?" I walked out; the nurse was standing right outside the door. She said, "I heard what he said, what do you want me to do?" I told her, "I want him out of the room; I don't know how." She said "I do. I'm calling Security. Since the problem Debra had before with him, we hover around the room when he's there."

When Tim kept up the sneering comments, Jeremy got up from the other bed and pulled him by the nape of his collar and was dragging him down the hall to the elevator. He put him in the elevator, pushed the Lobby button and said, "Don't come back." A few minutes later, two Security staff entered Debra's room. The tall male Security, whispered, "Where is he?" I told them what happened and he said, "I'll deal with him in the Lobby." When he pushed the button for the elevator, there he was; he had come back! The Security man took him by the arm and said "Oh no, we're going back down." The female Security asked what had happened, and the nurse was there to corroborate my story.

I sat next to Jerr and held his hand, and I prayed, "Please, God, help me deal with this." A phrase I had used in my seminars came into my mind, "There are some people who always seem angry and continuously look for conflict or try to manipulate it. Walk away, the battle they are fighting isn't with you, it is with themselves." Oh, God, how true, and how pathetic for Tim all these years!

Before I leave this rendition of the hospital, during the three days we were there, Sister Jeanette kept coming in with her prayer book. She told us she was going to pray for Debra. We immediately bowed out heads, and I clasped my hands. Sister reverently said, "Debra, I'm going to talk to you ." Then she read beautiful passages from the Psalms and then from the other parts of the Bible — passages that I had heard all my life and prayed from my own Bible. I was in tears. Then Sister fervently told Debra, "It's OK that you leave us, Debra, you're going to Jesus who is waiting for you. Walk toward the light. See the light and walk toward it." Then she would raise her eyes and look to see if there was a change in Debra. No — Debra continued gasping for breath. Sister would wait a few more minutes, then stood and told us, "I'll be back."

Hours later, she would return and the same scenario was repeated, and she would tell Debra, "Debra, your family is here, they love you, you have no more pain, it's OK to leave — to walk into the arms of Jesus." She would lift her eyes and….. no, no change in Debra's breathing.

Several more times, this routine was repeated and…… no change in Debra's breathing. Finally, Sister Jeanette came in and said she was leaving for the day and that she would be back in the morning and that she would remember Debra in her evening prayers. We thanked her. and she very slowly turned and walked out of the room with just a whisper of her shoes on the tile.

12:30 a.m., Wed. —

It was at this time that Jeremy and Donna had stepped out to the hall to use their cell phones. I believe Jeremy was calling his father. Donna was calling Lisa? Both Jerr and I moved to the side of Debra's bed, and I began stroking her arms and face — her skin was luminescent and soft — and her pixie cap of hair was silky — and we were saying *"We love you, sweetheart. We love you. You are so beautiful. May God take you from my arms into His arms and protect you for us always. Debra, we're here, sweetheart! We're here, your buddy Jerr and me! We know how much you've suffered we want to take this suffering from you and put it on us. We're so sorry, we're so sorry and we love you always!"*

2/22/12, Wed. -1:00 a.m. —

All of a sudden Debra flickered open her cloudy, but beautiful hazel eyes for a moment for the first time in three days and looked up at me. Her eyes closed! Then she stopped breathing. It was so silent! I waited for another gasp! There was nothing! I cried out, "Debra, no, no, no!" I waited a few seconds. Jerr who was now standing by me, holding Debra's hand, leaned over my shoulder and touched her face and hair. He put his arm around me and said, "She's gone, sweetheart, she's gone!"

I buzzed for the nurse, waited a second, then ran out of the room calling "Jeremy, Jeremy", and I started to run down the hall to the nurses' station, but they were already rushing toward us. I told them "My daughter! My daughter has stopped breathing!"

Donna and Jeremy had run back into the room. I heard Jeremy crying out, and Donna, too. When we all walked back into the room Jeremy was sitting on Debra's left side again and Donna on her right. They were holding her hands on each side of the bed and crying. Jeremy continued holding his Mom's hand and bent over them. After a couple of minutes, the nurse put her hand on Jeremy's shoulder and quietly said, "Jeremy, I have to check your Mom's heart." He moved barely to the side, never letting go. The nurse listened to Debra's chest, then to the left side of her neck and stood up and nodded her head twice at the other nurse in the room and looked at her watch. She turned to us and then to Jeremy and Donna and told us, "I'm so sorry! I'm so sorry! You can have all the time you want. She was a fighter! She fought very hard!" We were sobbing and hugging each other. My heart was pounding!

It was so silent in the room after the days and nights of her gasping and raspy breathing. The silence was horrible!

Jeremy lifted her blanket, took out a note he had written and put it on Debra's chest. He had also taken a photo of their hands clasping. The note read:

> "Mom, one of the last things you told me was that
> you wanted earrings. We had fun having our time
> getting ready for Florida, and you always told me

you wanted diamond earrings for the trip, so for
you I'm giving you one of mine, Love, Jeremy."

He had taken one of his black and white diamond earrings and
punched it through the paper and laid it under her blanket. Now
he told us he wanted it left with her at the hospital and then at the
funeral home and that it should be buried with his Mom. (*Much
later, we all convinced Jeremy that even if that's what he wanted to do,
it would be wiser to keep it for someone special in his life some day. He
finally agreed.*)

Then he and Donna walked out into the hallway where they were
both making phone calls. Much later when Lisa and Doug came
back to the hospital, Lisa walked up to the nurse in the hallway and
said "Tim would like to say his final goodbye." The nurse said "I
have to have Lorraine's permission." I said, "No, he already pulled
that this afternoon to get back in her room for a 'final goodbye' ".
The nurse said, "This afternoon, Debra was still alive and now she's
gone. He's lost a daughter, too. It will only be for a few minutes
and we'll be right next to him." So I agreed and we stepped across
the hall to the small waiting room. The nurse, Lisa and Doug and
Tim went in. Once again he got what he wanted. When they came
out, Lisa told Donna, "Come on, we'll take you home." and the
four of them left.

2:00 a.m. —

I called my sister, Chickie, and then Terri in Florida, and told them
"She's gone! Debra is gone! She just died!" Jerr called his brother,
Mark, and told them. Donna called Chris. Jeremy made the rest of
the calls.

Jerr and I remained with Debra. I didn't want to leave her. She
looked so beautiful, like she was asleep except her mouth was
open slightly. I wanted to lift her up and hold her in my arms but
I couldn't move her. She was already rigid. I kept stoking her face

and hair and telling her how much we loved her. How much we always loved her. I was sobbing. Jerr was holding me.

A supervising doctor in a starched, white coat then walked in and told us, "I have to confirm the nurses' report." She, too, listened to Debra's heart and side of her neck.

She asked: Is there anything I can do? Is there anything I can help you with?

I told her, "We don't know what to do! What happens now?"

Doctor: "She (She? She?) will remain here until the Release Certificate is prepared. She will go downstairs where she will be washed and be readied for release. The funeral home has to be contacted first thing in the morning and we can release her then."

The doctor asked about organ donation. We told her Debra had mentioned donating her organs to RPCI. The doctor responded that they don't take donated organs. (What — they don't want to see what they've done?) The doctor added: "She had a very strong heart. If that's your wish, she has to be taken down as quickly as possible." We said, "No!" In my heart, the thought crossed my mind that I didn't want to subject Debra to any more mutilation and pain! My intellect told me this was not a rational thought!

We spent another half hour with Debra; we didn't want to leave her, and I told Jerr, " I don't want Debra to be left alone. I want to stay with her. I want to lay next to her and wrap her in my arms." He just had his arms around me.

Then the nurse came in and asked if she could empty Debra's closet and give us her clothes and shoes — which she did and put them in a bag and handed it to me. (I guess that was our sign that we were to leave?) Jerr reached out and took the bag and with this arm around me, he nudged me out the door. We slowly walked down the hall, into the elevator and out the front entrance of the hospital. I passed the chapel, hesitated a moment and wanted to go in

— but I couldn't. What would I say to God, to Jesus now?! "Thanks a lot?" How could I convey the feelings I felt? Who was to blame? Who decided my daughter instead of me? Did we bear some of the fault, some of the guilt? Could we have done more? Could we have insisted that she seek another opinion no matter how it affected her feelings? Why was she made to suffer so much? Was it already too late back in 2009? Who....... What....... ???? In the car, I pounded the steering wheel until Jerr reached over and held my hands.

When Debra finally did leave us, it was shortly after the "negative influence" (*her father*) had left the room, and when Debra (*or Jesus*) decided it was her time and on her terms! During Debra's life, you could never tell her what to do but guide her in a way that when she did finally make a decision, it was because it was her own decision! Jeremy is very much like her in this respect. He's obedient, but he wants to make his own decisions, and we feel this adds to his maturity far beyond his age of sixteen.

I repeat that if we said the wrong thing to others during this time, or didn't know what to do, or didn't say the right thing, it's because we — and people in general — just don't know how to act in such a situation. They are frozen in a fog. It is all strange and foreign to us. We are not taught "social" skills in such a situation. I was only focused on Debra and not anyone else. It's very hard to know what to do. I can't even remember what people said.

Donna's version: "Sister Jeanette is the one who came in and told Debra that she was dying, and she was so rude to her, Mom. Then the other nurse, who really hurt her feelings, told her, "You are dying, you'd better face it!" And then that nurse was the one falling all over you and Jerry when you got there. What a phony!

"Mom, we were going to ask Hospice for a hospital bed so Debra would come home with me. I would spend my days and nights watching her and seeing to whatever medical treatment she needed. Debra told me, 'They won't let me have my IV and what I don't want is to gasp for breath or to starve to death.' Mom, there was no nutrition in her IV, only liquid to keep her hydrated; she WAS starving. The nurse said without nutrition, she would only have a couple of days. She told me she had cancer in her; Jeremy was sitting by her bedside holding her hand and crying and just looking at her. I barely heard what the doctors told Debra on that day. I was just outside her room, Mom. *(Wasn't this even a different version of what we had been told?)*

"Also, Ginny wanted the new PJs back that she had just given Debra, and we could not find them in her hospital room. Lisa had taken them and we asked her to return them. (It was weeks before they were returned.) Lisa was going to lend Jeremy Colton's suit and a suit for dad for the funeral. They never got them, never got them until the day before and they didn't fit. Jeremy was told to rent one at a tuxedo place.

2/22/12, 2:30 a.m. —

Jerr and I had left the hospital and were almost five miles away at the Grand Island Bridge just about to go through the toll booths when the nurse called and told us that she had just found Debra's black fur jacket. Could we return in the morning and pick it up? *(Black fur jacket? At the hospital?)*

I said "No, we're not that far away and it would be easier to get it now." So we went through the toll booth, took the first exit, and re-crossed the bridge to return to Lewiston and the hospital. *(All the way back, I prayed "Please, God, don't let us see her face covered up with a sheet. Please, God, please, don't let the room be empty."* But when we were unable to enter the locked main entrance, we had to go around to the Emergency Room entrance. The tall security guard — the one who had removed Tim before — already had her jacket in a bag and said "I'm very sorry for your loss." I told him, "Thank you for your help before." *(She had worn her best fur jacket to the hospital? Always it was a padded sports jacket she wore or a thermal jacket — but her fur jacket? I was shaking with chills. Why had she decided to do this?)*

On the way back to Williamsville, we again saw that Tim Horton's was open! We stopped for hot chocolate and donuts. I looked out the window and saw the Colucci Funeral Home right next door so then I knew where we needed to go in the morning. We arrived back in Williamsville about 4:30 a.m.

2/22/12, Wed., 6:00 a.m. —

Later, Donna told me that Debra (crying) said, "Don't tell dad and Jeremy you're leaving; she wrote a "Bucket List", and said what I don't want is to starve to death. She wanted her IVs back; she didn't want not to be able to breathe; the doctor never came back in to talk to her.

2/22/12, Wed. —

At home, we just fell on top of the bed. Jerr had just closed his eyes; I was awake and crying. At 7:30 a.m., the phone rang. Half asleep, Jerr jumped up: "It's Debra!" and went to answer the phone! It was Mark wanting to know if we wanted to meet them for breakfast. We told him that we had to go to the funeral home first thing. When Jerr hung up, he and I just held each other and sobbed and sobbed.

I cried out (and don't know how I had the audacity to say this), "Damn you, God, why did you have to listen to Debra and not to me?! Why did You have to listen when my daughter cried, 'I can't do this anymore. I can't do this anymore.' Why, oh why — with all Your power and might and sending Jesus to heal us and forgive our sins, why is there so much pain and cancer and loss in this world. Why can't there be a cure for cancer — You have the power! Why did You take my daughter and not me? And if You were going to take her anyway in the end, why was she made to suffer so much — be in so much pain? We were so hopeful in all the prayers and petitions and what doctors were saying. She has so much to live for — her son who she loved unconditionally and with his future goals. She is such a beautiful person, so creative in her art and gardens, so loving, oh, God, why?! Why?! Do people welcome death as a relief from the pain or do they fight to overcome the pain and live? God knows, she tried. She really tried because Debra, had a reason to live — Jeremy! Wasn't it important to you the kind of mother she was to her son?!

Then I remembered a phrase: "God understands our prayers even when we can't find the words to say them. Be at peace."

9:00 a.m.

We called Rob at Colucci Funeral Home. He was so calm and reassuring. I asked them what should we do? We didn't even know where to begin. Rob told us that if we came in, they would help us and answer all our questions. Thankfully, no one had ever been there to make any arrangements! Rob asked us did we decide to use them for the services? We told him, "Yes, definitely. We're coming to met with you." He gave us a 2:30 appointment.

11:00 a.m.

As we showered and re-dressed to go to the funeral home, Donna called that her father had told her, "I'm not going anywhere today, as a matter of fact; I'm going to be resting for the next two days!" Donna said, "Mom, we have to do this as soon as possible. I don't want my sister in that cold basement of the hospital. I want to see her! I don't want her to be alone!"

Chickie called and asked if there was anything she could do. I told her what we needed to do, and she wanted to go with us, so we drove to Tonawanda to pick her up, then picked Donna up in Niagara Falls.

Chickie: "When we were in the waiting room at the hospital with Donna, she said, "Amy, I know Aunt Lorraine might be mad that we never saw Debra except for once at their house in Williamsville when Debra first began her treatments. If you had told me what was happening , I wouldn't have ignored her. We'll get her a Mass card. I called Debra every month, left messages and finally when we didn't get any calls back, I thought she just doesn't want to hear from me."

I told her, "Don't think about it, Chickie, Debra just couldn't cope with more than one thing at a time and that was to fight for her life, and she was feeling so sick all the time. It wasn't that she didn't care for people, she just needed to do what she could for herself at this time in her life. I truly wished you had called me. By the same token, I could have called you, but we, too, were just going day to day with a hectic schedule. You know people don't always do the things properly during a time like this."

Then, "About Steve's illness, I have to live with what I did." She was referring to not realizing that a medication he was on had caused kidney disease.

2:30 p.m. —

I was dreading the visit to the funeral home, I was so terrified. My stomach was twisting and my heart pounding. I kept thinking, we have no business here to do this because of Debra — she was so full of life and happiness. But it is one of those things in life in which we have no choice. Rob helped us make the arrangements for my daughter's funeral. What would have been a horrible, nerve-wracking experience was tolerable with Rob's help. I felt calmer. Rob then told us, "Debra is already here; we picked her up this morning after I talked with you, and you confirmed that we were to make the arrangements. (*Oh, thank God, I cried twisting my hands! I wanted to see her! I wanted to say how sorry I was! I wanted to hold her, and kiss her, and say I wanted her to come home with us and to say a prayer over her! But that was not to be.*)

Rob then stated that we needed to decide on the selection of the casket. (I took a deep breath. *I was terrified all over again. A memory flashed back to thirty years before when my stepfather died suddenly on*

Christmas Eve in Colorado, and only Chickie, Debra and I could obtain
emergency seats on Christmas day on a fight to Denver and then connect-
ing to Colorado Springs. When we went to the funeral home there, we
were taken into a dimly-lit room with all the casket tops open and the
director pushing us in one room after the other, toward one casket after
another. All I felt was it was like a Frankenstein movie. I was terrified for
years!) But Rob handed us a beautiful, large 3-ring binder of caskets
in color from which to select Debra's casket. *(Thank God, again.)*

When we were given another book to select the prayer cards to be
used with the Guest Book, we bypassed all the religious symbols
and pictures and immediately selected ones with nature and those
that reminded us of the many areas she loved -- a winding path
across a bridge and into the woods (her favorite place to walk with
Jeremy); mountains (Colorado), sunset over an ocean (Florida and
Massachusetts), autumn leaves (New York and the woods in the
hills), waterfalls (Williamsville and Niagara Falls). When friends
saw the cards, they said, "OMG, this is so Debra. (The photo on her
prayer card was cropped from our "Women of Mary Kay" photo
shoot when the three of us were selected to the event.)

Finally, Rob asked us to list Debra's assets, bank accounts, savings
accounts, life insurance policy, property *(Nothing.)*. "How was she
supporting herself?" We were supporting her, and — just recently
Social Security Disability. Then he said, "Oh, then Social Services
will pay for the funeral. *(What?)* If she doesn't have any assets and
there's no life insurance, it will be Social Security. If it is later found
that she did have assets, then the responsibility for the entire cost
of the funeral and burial will have to be addressed." He outlined
the funeral home costs and the cost for the grave at the cemetery,
and referred us to their representative at the cemetery we chose. It
was the cemetery at the base of the hill where Debra took Jeremy
sledding! When we completed the arrangements and left, I thought
what a comforting experience especially when we have to endure
the horror of the unknown or the stories we've heard.

The four of us walked next door to Tim Horton's for coffee. I said, "I want to do a storyboard for Debra's funeral — "A Celebration of Life!" Instantly, we all had ideas. Chickie said we could get together at Amy's house tonight and work on them. We went to Office Max and purchased the boards, supplies and materials. Jerr was puzzled — a "storyboard"? I explained what some families do to highlight their loved one's life to those people who were not there over the years. Some people just have a favorite framed photograph and others do other things.

I spent the remainder of the afternoon pulling open all the photograph albums, going through boxes that hadn't been sorted, I was smiling and crying at the memories as the photographs recalled Debra's life. I thought that as we look at photographs from the past, we would never think that we would lose that person and especially lose someone to what Debra endured. Photographs are happy times, we smile, we pout, we act up, we pose, and the spirit of the person is revealed.

That evening at Amy's the ten of us worked on her large dining room table. We spent wonderful hours talking and working and pasting and cutting out, and arranging and rearranging but most of all remembering all our memories of Debra! Amy's three little girls wanted to help, too, and they took their sticker books out and used their stickers to add special memories to the storyboards — a crown (I always called Debra "Princess"), guitars, a "Rock Star" star; hearts, a skeleton face, butterflies, dolphins, flamingoes, palm trees, sandals, ice cream sundaes, little blue birds, a sun face, a moon (*Debra was a moon child and we always called each other on the full moon and promised to think of each other during the full moon no matter where we were*), and flowers, flowers, flowers. There was a section in the middle of one storyboard with a heart and Jeremy's pictures from birth to present with hearts, hearts, hearts.

On the word "LIFE" (of A Celebration of...) Amy created a zebra pattern — wow. It was so appropriate for Debra. OK, so it took her all night! But it was so Debra. And on the third storyboard, (with Jeremy's permission) we added Jeremy's note to his mom on the day she went to heaven and the photo of the two of them holding hands on that last day. This was all truly Debra! That was such a special night. Jerr sat on the living room sofa just watching us and later told me what a blessing it was to see families together like this, in spite of such sorrow. It was the first time he had experienced such a funeral preparation. How special and comforting it was to see all of us doing something happy for Debra. (Jewish tradition is when the loved one dies, they must be buried the same day, if possible, before sundown. If not possible, then before sundown the following day, except if it is the Sabbath, then they have no choice but to wait until the Monday. There are no open caskets, just a pine box, no wakes, and no bereavement meals. After the funeral, if the family wishes, they have a Shiva, there has to be twelve men, facing east, to say prayers at sundown. The Shiva is for three to seven days; the family provides a small buffet each day.)

That night, when we got home, I just paced the floor. I walked into the den and there were the hospital bags with Debra's last possessions. I sobbed and sobbed with all the memories circling my head and pounding in my heart. I prayed to God and felt only a silence.

I cried out to Debra: *"Oh, sweetheart, where are you?! Who are you with?! Did anyone come to get you in their arms?! Who would there have been to do that? Is there really an afterlife? Is it true that angels do not look like our depiction of angels on Christmas cards? Are they really big balls of light that float and carry nothing but immense love and warmth? I hope so, sweetheart, because I don't want you to be alone! I don't want you to be afraid! I don't want you to be in a place where I can't help you! I don't want you to be terrified about the unknown! I want to know that I will one day see you again and hug you with all my might! All we can rely on is the faith with which we were raised and the belief that there is a almighty God who watches over us and sends His emissaries (angels) to help us, and Jesus who came that we might one day be saved. For this I pray in His name."*

2/23/12, Thurs. —

I had told Debra's great aunt, Tia Connie about Tim (I was crying with anger!) and she in her wisdom said, "You're a better woman than he is a man. Let it roll off your back. You have a great husband who loves you and that is your strength. Believe in that, Lorrie. Your daughter still needs you. It's not finished yet." "Tia, I remember someone's father once said: The higher a circus monkey climbs a pole, the more his ass shows!" Now we were laughing!

2/23/12,

My brother, Frankie, from New Mexico called. "We love you, Lorrie and we love Debra, we will be praying for her."

2/23/12 —

My younger sister in Colorado — Erma's email: "God can only give you the burdens you can carry, but how does he know what a mother can bear?"

(Remember that their son, Aaron, died with leukemia at age 25, two weeks after his daughter was born. Erma, too, would sit in his hospital room and email the day's progress, treatments or setbacks. Erma and I had kept in close contact throughout these three years. She knew what we were going through. She has done so much for Debra through the American Cancer Society and Compassionate Friends. In my angry moments, I would wonder how all these activities help — the races, the pinky, pinky stuff and gimmicks, the fundraisers, constant solicitations for funds with the letters becoming shorter and shorter and not outlining their accomplishments, just "send us the money", the petitions, the prayers, the candles, the walks, etc. etc. And then the answer comes, it doesn't help the dead, it helps the living.....and keeps the deceased in our memories.)

2/23/12 —

When I told my Florida friend, Sue, how broken up we were, especially Jerr, she counseled me to have both of us, especially

Jerr, write down memories of Debra, whatever he can think of. Keep them in a Memory Book. (*I remembered all the notes I had taken through the years of every conversation I had with the girls and especially when Debra had her first surgery and was diagnosed with cancer and how these notes have become this book.*)

2/23/12 —

My cousin from California, Carla, and her son, Colton: Gave her condolences and told us, "If there's anything you need, let me know. I mean anything! I have more than enough; I have more than I need and can help in any way. Debra is doing cartwheels in Heaven, free of pain! Please believe that!"

2/23/12 —

Chris called and told me about all the difficulties with Debra's father. "He's supposed to be an adult; had problems with the funeral director. Then he had a problem about Debra's proxy. The proxy does not have to be someone related by blood but by her chosen proxy; someone she trusts. Debra had said something about it's like paying a bill once a month; I don't want to hear anything more from him. He created all kinds of problems through the years with car repairs and payments and pulling tricks; just everything! All Jeremy hears is about money, money, money, arguments and the car he's been promised. It will never happen. Her father acts like a big game, but he talks shit. My payment is to do something special for Debra. I really loved her."

"I know, Chris. I know everything you've done for her, even in spite of your own problems and challenges. Nothing in anyone's life or family goes smoothly. You were the one there for her right from the beginning and to the end."

2/23/12 —

I called Lisa and left the message that when she's ready, we can make arrangements later to see about Debra's clothes, jacket, and jewelry, and anything she had left there. Chris was there; we didn't finish our conversation. (*Lisa never called back but gave Jeremy a box of his Mom's belongings. He told me, "Grandma, what am I supposed to do with this box of my Mom's things?". Jeremy, we'll decide later; not now; don't worry about it.*

2/23/12 —

From then on, our cell phone rang non-stop (we had disconnected our land line service when we left for Florida). When we would turn our cell phone off or charged it, we would find dozens of messages, and later people told us that the recorded message was that the inbox was full. People stopped by and wanted to bring food and other items. Tradition is that the family holds visitation hours or a bereavement luncheon. (*Thank you so much but really our refrigerator and pantry was empty, and we didn't know how long we were going to be here. Several of our family and friends were in Lewiston or Florida, or scattered across the United States.*)

2/23/12, 4:00 p.m. —

Rob from the funeral home called and said that Jeremy and his grandfather had been there. His grandfather had changed the casket selection (*as I knew he would*) and will pay the upgrade cost. Jeremy changed the clothing we had chosen for her — he wanted her to wear black because that's how he remembers her (black and white were her favorite colors). But when they saw the new clothes that Ginny had already dropped off, he changed his mind. Debra will wear the new small white jeans that she was so proud of, a beautiful white blouse and a lacy sweater both from Macy's that Ginny had delivered that morning. Donna also wanted Debra to have her new zebra blanket.

During the summer, Debra had informed me that she had given Lisa permission to throw away all her old clothes, torn, snagged, tights with the runs, too big, don't fit, out of style — all her old clothes. Debra told us that with her weight loss, she was going to buy all new clothes and shoes, and we had promised her a fun shopping trip. She had bought white jeans she wanted to bring to Florida; she was amazed she could fit into a 4 or 5. She had weighed 155 that summer and at the end, she was 120.

Jeremy's grandfather told him we were giving him $25,000 when Debra died! *(Where did that come from?)*

Donna wanted something simple for Debra, wanted Debra in her black sweater. "But everybody else made the decision, not what Debra told me she wanted!" she said.

5:00-6:00 p.m. —

The three of us were invited to Chickie's for dinner. Steve said, "Nothing fancy but I made tuna noodle casserole." "Nothing fancy" was oh, so good! After dinner, we again worked on the storyboards with Janet and Amy and the girls.

Chickie told us, "Lorr, did you notice when Tim left Debra's room, Debra felt at ease to give up her spirit?" *(Yes, I did.)* Chickie told me about one instance when she and Amy had gone to the small waiting room across from Debra's room, Donna told Jeremy, "Your grandmother is an amazing woman, she worked at Carborundum for twenty-five years, started the Festival of Lights, was a charter member of the NYS Seaway Trail. She was at the bottom and she picked herself up."

Chickie: "Don't worry about Tim at the funeral, there's lots of men around and Eric, Chris, Aaron, Steve, Bill, Jeremy, Phil — they won't let anything happen. We all said we would keep an eye out and surround you."

Donna: Mom, Ginny cut my hair for me and she offered to do your hair, too, but she saw that you have it done professionally. She didn't charge me for the hair cut, but these men here piss me off, they come over here, no shirts or borrowed suits from Lisa, were told to go to Tuxedo and rent them. Why? Dad is dropping Jeremy off at Gander Mountain as he had to go bowling with friends. He didn't bring any pictures! Phil is a phony. We had two different priests and dad told me we picked the wrong one!

"Donna, do you realize that Jeremy going bowling with his friends, is like all of us at Amy's and Chickie's house. We laughed, we cried, we worked, and put something special together for Debra. Jeremy's inner circle — his fifteen closest friends — will help him deal with what he's feeling, and it is not an inappropriate thing for a teenager to do. He must be feeling lost. Who is he going to be with tonight — his father, his stepmother, his stepsisters — none of who could care less about Debra. Can you imagine them sitting around mourning Debra? Fat chance! If it was my decision, I would have moved Jeremy in here with us until after the funeral, and he would have shared with our family, and I would have had the opportunity to explain what had happened at the end and what was going to happen for the funeral and burial. He needs to be with someone who can give him attention, affection and love — and if his friends can do that, then so be it."

2/24/12, Fri. —

I was very uneasy with the upcoming funeral service. I didn't want any problems, and I didn't want the service for Debra to be spoiled with a scene. I didn't know what to do. I called Rob at the funeral home and told him what happened with Debra's father on the two occasions at the hospital. He said, "I'm so glad you told me. We've encountered such experiences before with families. We'll have some of our directors on the day of the funeral, and if he causes trouble all you have to do is come to the door, nod at us, and we will discreetly handle it." I was so grateful for his help!

2/24/12 —

Debra, I did what you wanted, sweetheart. I found your friend, Greg, after all these years, and told him what you said and how you wanted him to know how special he was in your life. He said "Oh my gosh, it's so funny that you would call! Just the other day, my wife, Kim, and I were

going through some unopened boxes since our move, and we found Debra's
photo album. Give me your address and I'll mail it to you."

A gift: I went out shopping for clothing and shoes for the funeral for both
Jerr and me as we didn't have the appropriate outfits here. Jerr called me
and said Greg was bringing Debra's photo album over! His wife had said,
"You have to deliver it, Greg, if you mail the package, it will be too late."
When Greg came over, did you see, Debra, how we spent forty minutes
together? He has grown into quite a mature young man, with a wife and
four children — can you imagine?! He said they were very involved in
their church on Grand Island and that his wife would have been happy
to invite Debra to dinner — that's the kind of person she is. God bless
her! We looked through your photo album and you had written notes on
every page. Later, I took it to the funeral home and everybody was looking
through it. So many happy memories of years ago, sweetheart, and all
your cute comments, and I was reminded how you looked at miracles
as 'gifts'.

2/25/12 —

After dinner at Chickie's, we worked again on Debra's storyboards.
*(Phrases kept wafting through my mind: "I love you, Mummy." "I love
you, too, Debra!"*

2/26/12, Sun., 2-4 p.m. —

Debra's funeral services.

We arrived at the funeral home too early — about 1:00 p.m. — and
we and Donna stopped at Tim Horton's for a hot chocolate and
then over to the funeral home. Chickie and Steve had parked
right next to us, and we all went in. Rob was there to greet us and
showed us into the appropriate room. There was soft lights and
beautiful calming music, I saw the chairs set up and the beautiful
table with the Guest Book and Debra's prayer cards! Rob said
we would get the Guest Book tomorrow after her burial and any

envelopes that were left. We requested that "Amazing Grace" to be played at the appropriate time.

And then in the front of the room, was the casket and.......my daughter, Debra. I lost my breath and turned away. I didn't want to see her there...but I wanted to just pick her up and just hold her as I had done when she first came into my life. We put up the three storyboards of "A Celebration of Life" on tripods and opened Debra's photograph album on a small table at the entrance.

When we finally had the courage, we went up to the casket to see Debra. I was so anxious to see her but so frightened. She looked so beautiful, so peaceful, just like she was asleep, those long eyelashes once again sweeping her precious cheeks — not at all like she looked in the hospital. She was wearing, I assume, her new white jeans; we could see the white blouse and beautiful white sweater. Her short pixie hair was so soft and silky. I wanted to pick her up and hold her and never let her go. I was crying with pain, with sorrow, and heartbreak. Jerr was holding me.

People began arriving and we stepped to the back of the room to greet them. Jeremy and Phil came in, they were alone. I asked Jeremy if he wanted to go see his mom. "No, grandma, not yet." I told him, "She looks so beautiful and peaceful, just like she's asleep." I saw that he kept glancing over at the front of the room while he was looking at the storyboards and Debra's album and talking to people. Several minutes later, I saw Jeremy approach the casket on his own, and a few minutes later, Phil stood next to him. It was heart-wrenching. Jeremy looked so nice and neat and quite a young man.

Later, Rob told us he had wrapped a rosary around Debra's hands and that she would be buried with it. The cross that Jeremy had selected was beautiful, gold and ornate and displayed against the top. Rob said, "Does Jeremy get that back?" *Yes.* When Chris and his boys came in, he put his guitar pick in Debra's hands.

Donna's father who kept circling the room, went to the kneeler and was hunched over the casket, mumbling the same way he did in the hospital room. The floral drape arrangement that we and my sister's family had ordered was beautiful and colorful, just like Debra. It had an array of several different flowers — it reminded us of all the gardens she had designed.

(I remembered again the garden at Chris' house. Then we thought back to Father's Day 2011 when Debra planted "Deb's garden" for Jerr's Father's Day.)

2:00 p.m. —

Friends and relatives started coming in; some we hadn't seen in years and some we didn't know at all, but they were there for her. *(Debra, did you see all the love — the love that was yours spread out over the years was all in one place?!)*

My nephew, Tommy, who I hadn't seen since he was a younger boy, came and hugged me. I introduced him to Jerr, and he said, "I see you've finally got a good man." I said, "He is a gem, a perfect person, and I am so lucky with him." He said, "I can see that." We caught up briefly on his family's news.

Then Tommy looked over and asked, "How has 'he' been?" I explained a little bit of what been happening. He told me how his father (Tim's brother) had died and about some of his medical problems, and that he hasn't talked to his mother or her second husband in six years. I told him, his sister, Cathy, had posted a message on the obituary page. We were so grateful.

Father Michael came up to me and we talked for a few minutes. Jeremy had heard me say that when the priest comes in, he would say a few prayers and then it would be the last time we see Debra. He went up to the kneeler and stayed there, just looking at Debra, and then crying; all of us were crying when they saw him. Phil came up and I was on the other side. Father told us, "There's no hurry; I'll wait." Finally, Jeremy started to stand up, and I introduced him to Father Michael and Father started the prayer service. And "Amazing Grace" was played.

After the prayers, Rob announced that people from the back of the room could came up first, pay respects to the family and could walk by to see Debra for the last time. I just sat clutching my hands and can't even remember who came by. One by one as people left, we then had private time with Debra; I stroked her soft hair again and said *"Goodbye, my sweetheart, daughter. May you rest in peace. I love you, sweetheart."* (*And I heard a soft, "I love you two, too!?"*)

Jeremy didn't want to leave. He was still sitting on the loveseat in front of his Mom, just looking at his mother. Rob said, "He can take all the time he needs; no problem." The large room was empty and still Jeremy sat — alone.

As we waited at the back of the room, Chickie, Donna and I began taking down the storyboards and packing up our bags with the photo album and other items. After about 20 minutes, we left to pack the car. When we returned to the room, Jeremy had said goodbye to his mother and was leaving with his father.

Chris had been waiting for me and came up and said, "Meet me at my car, Lorraine. I have some jewelry and other items from Debra that I want to give you." Tim and Donna had left the room about five minutes before us, but they remained parked next to us in the handicapped section. We don't know where they went afterward, but Chickie heard one of the friends say something to Donna who replied, "Let me go home and change and I'll meet you."

Chickie, Steve, Jerr and I went to the Olive Garden for dinner and ran into Amy and family and we hosted the mini-bereavement dinner together.

At 1:40 p.m. —

Tia Connie, sobbing, had left a message on our cell phone, "Let me give you some advice, daughter, you stand there with a smile on your face because your little girl is in a better place. Let everybody see your strength and faith. She is at peace! She is not in pain!"

Jerr asked me to post his message on Debra's Guest Book, and it was then I saw the other messages of kind people and friends, and my former executive and his wife, a beautiful and inspirational Christian couple and family! They were examples of moral, ethical, principled people, and it was my privilege and blessing to work with them. I began my college education when I typed the reports for their three kids!

M.J. Colucci & Son Funeral Chapels	*Guest Book for Debra Lynn Lafornia (Died February 22, 2012)*
Bonum and Janet Wilson *Charleston, SC 29412 March 11, 2012 10:09 PM*	*So sorry to hear of the death of your daughter, Debra. Our thoughts and prayers are with you and all your family, Sincerely, Janet and Bonum*
frankie & sarah lee chavez *santa fe, nm February 26, 2012 11:04 AM*	*oh what a beautiful angel we all have to look over us now — makes us remember to be together in all our thoughts and actions — we are all blessed for the past knowing Debra and from now on sharing her.*
SEREDA BLUM *HOLLYWOOD, FL* *February 25, 2012 2:32 PM*	*Dear Lorraine and Family, Words cannot express how sorry and sad I am with the passing of Debra. I am so happy that I got to meet her and Jeremy. Her smile was so, so special-she was so happy to be in Florida and so happy that Jeremy was having so much fun. My love and prayers are with you all. Love, Sereda*
Jerry *Williamsville, NY* *February 25, 2012 10:15 AM*	*For all the time I knew you, I loved you. I waited every day for your funny phone calls and when I teased and gave it back to you, you laughed and laughed. You were a joy to me and your mother. Jerry*
Connee & Nick Safis *Antioch, California* *February 24, 2012 2:07 PM*	*We loved you, Deb, may you rest in peace. Uncle Nick and I will remember your infectious laugh and loving ways she died too young. God bless her*

2/27/12, Sunday, 1:00 a.m. —

Darling Debra, you looked so beautiful and peaceful today, and for an instant, I thought, OK stop joking and wake up. We need you, sweetheart. But, of course, I knew Tia was right, you didn't need the pain you had endured. The service was so simple and yet elegant and not morbid or sad with people sobbing over you — something you said you never wanted, although we were all in tears. Did you see all your family and friends coming together? Why does it take a tragedy like this to bring people together? Did you see how grown up Jeremy was when he stood or knelt next to you? And then he became your little boy and cried. Phil had bought Jeremy dress pants and a white shirt, and he looked so nice. Lisa gave me the "Bucket List" which you had written in your last days. It was all about Jeremy. Lisa asked Rob to make a copy of it. I promise to fulfill it to the best of my ability. I read where Jeremy promised you that he would graduate, and I promise you that you will be there with us when he does. Goodbye, my precious little girl, we love you, we'll miss you and you were a joy to us always. May you be with God and Jesus and be there when we come.

Fr. John Mahony, a retired U.S. Army Colonel who survived the 19th floor of the North tower of the World Trade Center on 9/11/01, who recited the Lord's Prayer while descending the smoky stairs and suddenly he felt wonder, God's peace and Christ's love is all around us. "I know with a certainty that I will rise from this shell like a child fresh and clean from a bath, and I will be wrapped in the warmth of his love and his forgiveness and His peace." I remembered this again.

Donna: "Mom, Debra had told me what she wanted done and what she wanted to wear. When I saw what Jeremy and dad had picked out for her, it was totally inappropriate. Thank goodness, they changed their minds when they saw what had already been picked out for her to wear. Why did everybody else get involved when Deb had told me what she wanted?!"

2/27/12, Monday, 12:30 p.m., —

The burial services in Lewiston, NY.

The director had opened the little chapel in the English Tudor building, and then asked some of the men to act as pallbearers — Phil, Chris, Jeremy, Colton, one of the staff and himself. We were seated in the chapel for a few minutes and then Debra was brought in. Her beautiful flowers covered the top of the casket. Another priest, Father Michael, recited readings and words of farewell, then one of the Colucci staff again asked people in the back to come forward, lay a hand on the casket and say goodbye to Debra for the final time. (NO! NO! NO!) Chris came up; he was really broken up, and I held onto his hand and said "Don't leave, Chris, you belong with our family." Donna, Jerry and I were in the front row. I was holding their hands.

We sat in the chapel until we were informed Debra was at her gravesite. Jerr and I were first asked to stand by her side. I saw that the location was by a lovely tree and looked up at the hill where she always took Jeremy sledding in the winter and the woods where they walked. I was clutching Jerr's hand so hard and said that I said I couldn't watch her lowered into the ground! I felt that then it would be final. We turned away and sat in the car sobbing. I saw that the rest of the group were then taken to the site and they watched as the casket was lowered and then they turned away. I didn't want to leave. I didn't want to leave her out there — all alone.

A poem by Barbara Winter came to my mind:
When you come to the edge of all the light you know
And are about to step off into the darkness of the unknown,
Faith is knowing one of two things will happen:
There will be something solid to stand on, or you will be taught how to fly.

My sweetheart, Debra, may you have peace....free of pain....free of worries....free of the weights that keep us bound on this earth....and may you fly to heights unknown to us ordinary humans, into the hands of God....until we meet again. We love you always. I heard the whisper of the breeze through the trees, I love you two, too!

Chickie, Steve, Janet and Amy and the three of us met at the Como, and we had a wonderful spicy Italian lunch.

That evening, exhausted, we fell into bed and slept for twelve hours.

2/28/12, Tues., 3:00 p.m.

Donna called and said Jeremy and Dad and Lisa had gone to her father's house. Phil dropped Jeremy off at 8:30 p.m. last night in Tonawanda. Jeremy had decided to wash clothes at the last minute and his clothes were not dried.

Donna's version: "Mom, Debra didn't want that "muscle relaxer" shot, and she informed Sister Jeanette. I was outside the room. I heard what the doctor said. I went back in when he left; Debra and I hugged and she cried, 'Donna, I don't want to die.' Chris came in after work and said he'd stay with her, so I left the hospital to go shower and change. When I came back later that afternoon, Debra was already asleep." *(We have never been able to determine what the "muscle relaxer" was that she was given. All requests for her medical records have come to naught. To this day, we have never received them from any facility. When we ask, other doctors/friends are as puzzled as we are.)*

2/28/12, Tues. —

During our nightly calls with Terri, she informed me that at the general members meeting of the local political party (*of which we are both officers*), Alan, the president, announced what had happened to Debra, and there was a moment of silence for her. His wife, Shelly, was crying and so was Ellen, the Program Chairman. Terri says to me, "The more you talk about it, the more you heal;

you never lose the sadness. I know that was so when I lost my mother two years ago."

2/29/12, Wed. — 2:00 a.m.

I couldn't sleep; so I unpacked Debra's clothing from in the hospital bag we were given. When I saw Debra's clothing, I hugged them to my heart and just sobbed and sobbed until I couldn't breathe or sit up. She had worn to the hospital her best tights, her new "Hard Rock, Hollywood" glitter t-shirt, her favorite sneakers, there was her black soft leather wallet with all her ID, several dollars and change. Jeremy's picture was in the middle section where she saw it every time she had to produce her ID and the doctor's cards. I could see every time she carried it and used it. Then there was her black fur jacket. *Why, God? Why had she felt the need to wear her best clothes to the hospital? Why?* OMG!

Exhausted, I couldn't sit still so I did what I do best — make lists.

-Pay the funeral home.

-Call Social Security and inform them.

-Call Phil with the instructions from Social Security for Jeremy since he would receive the $255 burial fee and the monthly benefits from her account until he's 18 years of age or until he graduates. SSA outlined the line of succession is surviving spouse (none) and then minor children

-Cancel Debra's cell phone account. The rep informed me that her signed contract would be closed and that the other three phone numbers on her account would not be affected. I called Phil to inform him of this, and he told me, "No, Jeremy is on Tim's cell phone account." "Not true, Phil, it was Debra's account." He will notify Tim. (What I was told by Verizon was totally incorrect; the cell phone company cancelled all the phone numbers!)

-Notify the Department of Motor Vehicles.

-Notify her auto insurance agent.

-Call our attorney for a copy of Debra's will since Chris could not find it. I requested that Jeremy receive a copy of it also.

Chris called and said he had asked Lisa every day for Debra's jewelry that he had given her over the years (jewelry of black diamonds and white diamonds — a ring, a pendant, and earrings). He didn't want them back, but he wanted me to save them for Jeremy's wife. Lisa never gave them to Chris. I informed Phil and asked him if Lisa had given Jeremy her jewelry and that Debra wanted me to hold it. Phil: "I have no problem with that."

Phil said he had the jewelry.

L: Phil, did Lisa give you her clothes?

Phil: I don't know what was in the bag she gave Jeremy.

2/29/12, Wed. —

When I spoke to Phil; he was abrupt and short with me (*Was he at work or was someone listening on the other end?*). He hardly said anything but acknowledged that he had received the will.

I informed Phil about the conversation with Social Security and when I started giving him the information, he said there's a SSA office near here, I'll take Jeremy there. He was interested when I said Jeremy was going to get $255 Death Benefit and then monthly checks until he was 18 or until he graduated. SSA would not take Jeremy's information on the phone and that they needed to see him and his documents.

3/5/12, Mon. —

Donna went to the cemetery with flowers for Debra; she had taken a rose and a carnation from her casket drape to try to dry them. Donna goes to the cemetery almost every day. Jerr tells her "He's very impressed at her commitment to caring for Debra's grave. We go there about once a week because of the distance, but she's done a really nice job; making sure the flowers are watered; weeds taken out; grass will be growing in the spring, we hope.

Today I thought of one of the gifts I had received when I made Curcillo twenty years before — *"A butterfly lights beside us like a sunbeam. And for a brief moment, its glory and beauty belong to our world. But then it flies on again, and though we wish it could have stayed longer, we feel so lucky to have seen it."* With my love and gratitude, Fr. Ken+

3/12/12, Mon. —

I spoke to Jeremy today, and he said Lisa had given him a box of Debra's clothes, shoes.

J: Grandma, can we talk about what she gave me?

L: *Did she give you any jewelry, Jeremy?*

J: Yes.

L: *What did she give you?*

J: A black diamond and white diamond ring, black diamond and white diamond cross, black diamond and white diamond cross, silver chains, and another diamond something.

L: *These were all gifts to your mom from Chris, and he wanted them back only to give them to us to keep for you, Jeremy.*

Note: Jeremy said he'll bring them with him when he comes to Florida in April. (*He did.*) We will keep them for him until the appropriate time with the other gold and diamond ring from Chris' grandmother that Chris also gave Debra. *These items, plus the small amount of savings she had for Jeremy constituted her "estate" — all her worldly goods, a collection of a life time — could be held in a handkerchief. She left this world as she came into it with nothing and wrapped in a blanket.*

3/12/12, Mon. —

Donna went to the gravesite today. Debra's marker isn't here yet, but she looked at the other markers, and there won't be room for the poem she wrote. All the markers have just the name, the birth year and the year of death. (*We were told by the cemetery director this because of increasing identity theft!*)

"Mom, when Ziggy comes with me, he goes and sits under the tree and doesn't want to leave. He looks so peaceful like Deb is stroking him like she always did. The director has given me permission to allow Ziggy out of the car because he sees how I take care of him."

March 2012 —

Jerr and I remained in Williamsville for one and a half months finalizing as much as possible all of Debra's financial affairs. When we returned to Hollywood, Donna made our reservations for us and gave us her Jet Blue voucher credit, her gift to us. (A year earlier Donna had paid for a flight to Las Vegas for her and Debra, a trip cancelled due to Debra's hospitalization.)

We returned to a hundred more cards, memorials, trees planted in our friend, Stanley's forest in Israel — so many thoughtful and charitable gifts. I began the task of acknowledging each one — over 200 not only from here but from my friends in England — mailing the note with Debra's prayer card.

Then in several conversations, everyone agreed that Jeremy needed to keep his trip plans to go to Florida. (*I prayed that Debra could see how independent he was and that she was watching over him.*)

4/5-12/12 - Fri. to Fri. — Jeremy's visit with us! 🛬 🛬

4/6/12, Fri.

Jeremy had a horrendous flight experience on Spirit Airlines. Passengers were informed to be at the airport by 9:00 p.m. for the 11:30 p.m. flight. The plane didn't depart Niagara Falls until 2:30 a.m. (2:30 a.m. vs. 11:30 p.m.?). Earlier we had paid for a seat upgrade with more space than the cramped leg room on regular seats. He was happy to be in sunny Florida. When the plane was going to be delayed, Donna and Jeremy returned home as they only lived five minutes away from the airport, HOWEVER, they fell asleep, Donna's cell phone alarm did not go off, and when I called with a big smile at 2:00 a.m. to see if Jeremy had departed, I had awakened them! Donna screamed for Jeremy, and they dashed to the airport. His suitcases had already been checked. (*I prayed and told Debra to take care of her son if this trip was meant to be! Please don't let him be disappointed!*) Donna dropped Jeremy off and then went to park. It was 2:20 when she entered the terminal and saw that Jeremy had dashed through the security line and had boarded! "OMG, Mom! OMG!"

When we picked Jeremy up at the airport (finally!), we had to stop at McDonalds for breakfast.

He brought two wonderful thank you cards for me and Jerr, and a present from him that Debra had bought me for Christmas and never had the opportunity to send — a Kindle! In her last months of life, she was still thinking of others! She had mentioned to Donna she hadn't been able to get to the post office to mail my Christmas present to me. Donna went out and purchased $90 of gift cards from Amazon. Before we left Williamsville, Donna was supposed to give it to us and when she found out we had decided to return to Florida, she was so upset and wanted to get them to us, but there was a torrential rain storm that night and we didn't want her to chance driving to us to deliver it. So Donna packed it up for Jeremy to bring it on the plane. In Florida, he spent two days setting it up. Every time I hold the Kindle in my hands, Debra's spirit will be with me and prayers will go to the three of them — my two daughters and grandson.

We had planned a different itinerary for Jeremy's visit, and when we discussed it with him, he didn't say anything, but an hour later, he came back and said "Grandma, I would like to go to all the places I went with my mom, and can I still swim at night if we do that?"

So that's what we did,

4/7/12, Sat. — The Jungle Queen with a stop first for lunch at Bahia Cabana.

4/8/12, Sun. — Jeremy again woke up to his "surprise" Easter basket and lots of treats in it. Then we went to Easter Sunday Mass. *(Jeremy had to wear his cargo short and a casual shirt to church. His new dress outfit had been stolen at the Niagara Falls Airport at Spirit Airlines when Security (or someone there) must have opened his suitcase. Several grooming items were punched with holes. Thank goodness I had told him to pack personal grooming items in a plastic baggie. His brush/comb was broken in two. This did not happen in the baggage storage area!)*

We then had a "snackies" lunch, then went to Tropical Acres for dinner — steak dinners for the men and salmon for me.

4/9/12, Tues. —

We walked the Broadwalk at the ocean and went into all the souvenir shops, stopping for lunch at Rocco's Pizza which was Jeremy's choice — the aroma of fresh pizza as we walked by was the decider!

Later that evening, we went to the Hard Rock Café for dinner and Jeremy bought another souvenir T-shirt. From his savings, he purchased another T-shirt to bring back to a friend. We bought one for Donna.

4/10/12, Tues. —

To Aventura Mall where Jeremy bought a watch, and we replaced the Easter Sunday clothing — black dress slacks and white shirt

— the new outfit he had worn to the funeral. Then to the Anne Kolb Nature Center, climbed the stairs up to the tower and then back down to the wooden pathway to the water — like he and his mother did.

One evening, Jeremy and I were out at the pool deck and were standing at the railing overlooking the Intracoastal. We saw the planets Jupiter and Mars?? so clear in the sky, and I said the bigger, brighter one was his Mom and the smaller one was him. We quietly talked about illness and death, and all of a sudden, right below our feet, Jeremy heard a sound, and then saw four huge shadows appear in the water right along the wall where we were standing! Four manatees — two large ones and two small ones, popped out of the water, remained right below us, then slowly floated up the waterway and turned left into the canal! We were so excited. I told Jeremy how unusual it was to see even one manatee. In our nine years living there, we had seen them three times. As a matter of fact, my best friend, Sue, who lived seven floors higher, could spot them sooner than we could, and she would phone us — "Look, look." Sometimes we were lucky enough to be home and run to the balcony and sometimes we would just have the message on our phone when we returned home. (*Jeremy, that's your Mom's gift to us!*)

Returning home from Aventura Mall, Ocean Drive was completely blocked and police wouldn't let us pass to the half-block entrance to our condominium. Our residence is located across the street from The Westin Diplomat (remember that story?). We sat for over thirty-five minutes, then when we could take the left turn up onto the Intracoastal Bridge into Hallandale Beach, we made a U-turn, came back over the bridge and the policemen stationed at that intersection allowed us to get down the street into our garage — WHY? The president was speaking at The Diplomat.

When we got home, Jeremy and I went out on the balcony at the end of our 10th floor. We could look right into the side entrance of the hotel which was covered with two white tents into which the limousines drove. Outside there were snipers on the hotel roof overlooking the balconies of the condo right next door and probably across at the balconies in our building. There were 130 motorcycle police escorts, the fire department, an enormous white truck with black printing on the side — TERRORISM SQUAD — dozens of police cars, and after the few minutes that he was at the hotel fundraiser, this entourage drove up Ocean Drive a half mile away to Golden Beach (Millionaires Row) for a private fundraising reception at the home of one of the residents. Every other stop he made that day in the Miami/Hollywood area was publicized and covered — except this stop. Jeremy took photos of the happenings to post on Facebook.

Later in the week, it was good Debra was watching over us because on the Wednesday — two days before Jeremy returned home, I became ill at 2:30 a.m. I prayed, *Oh, God, not now, not with Jeremy here!* But at 7:30 p.m., I woke Jerr up and said I have to go to the hospital; I've been sick all night. Jerr said, "We have to wake Jeremy up." Jerr quietly called "Jeremy, wake up and get dressed; we have to take Grandma to the hospital." He was shocked but quickly got dressed and ready. When Jeremy came out of the bedroom, I looked at his face and saw shock and disbelief! I gave him a little smile and said "I'm sorry, sweetheart, but I'm not feeling well and have to go to the hospital."

With my directions, he drove me to the hospital! In the E/R, he still looked traumatized and my heart broke. I could imagine that he was thinking about his mother and I was very upset. About a couple of hours later, to distract him, I suggested that he and Jerr go to lunch at the McDonald's in the hospital. When they came back to the E/R, the doctor had already told me I was going to be admitted *(Oh, no, oh, no.)* When I was taken to my room, I drew Jeremy driving directions from the E/R back home. I did not want Jeremy driving during rush hour or at night so I told them to leave.

Later that evening when the guys called, they said they had stopped for pizza (*and I bet they didn't have fresh vegetable "snackies" with bleu cheese dip to go with the pizza!*) Jeremy kept calling me until almost 10:00 p.m., and I kept telling him I was OK, I was OK now that I was getting treated.

Jeremy and I had a talk about God, and he asked "Why do I keep losing the people I love. Why does God do these things to people?" I told him, "*It wasn't God; he's not a vengeful God. It's our own bodies that fail us and what we do to them that might cause us to get sick, or our environment, or any other number of things.*"

Jerr and Jeremy returned the next morning and again went to McDonalds for breakfast, and again at 2:30 I urged them to leave. I told Jeremy everything would be alright, and he said, "I know, Grandma." We said our goodbyes, and he held me so tight. I was sobbing so hard for this boy and gave thanks for his maturity and composure once he understood situations and for my husband who is a gem. The nurse came in worried about the activity on my monitor, and I just said I was upset. The guys stopped at the ocean because Jeremy had decided to buy souvenir t-shirts for his 10 friends; they had dinner at Rocco's.

Thursday: Although loaded to with taxes in her office, God bless my best friend, Terri, who took the time off and had already offered to help Jeremy get ready, pack, and take them to the airport, walk him through the security line up to the point where only ticketed passengers could go. They got to the airport at 7:00 p.m.; his flight was 9:30 p.m. Then Terri brought Jerr to the hospital, and he stayed with me until I was discharged four days later.

Jeremy's return fight on Spirit Airlines was another nightmare (again)! The 9:30 p.m. departure didn't happen. He was alone at the departure gate; the flight kept getting delayed; his cell phone was running out of power, because he had packed his charger for the "three hour" flight home. Then at one point he sent Donna a text that they had been put on a plane and then had to deplane and return back to the terminal! Donna kept calling me throughout the night, because I was in a panic. I told her how she could watch the status of his flight. She kept calling me that it still showed a big red "X". I did not know what we could do — how could I get to him at the airport, how could anyone get to him — Security wouldn't let them pass, I tried calling the airport to see if there was anyone who could help and got no answer, just pinch this number and punch that number. He is sixteen years old! Finally about 3:00 a.m., Donna saw the website message flash "In Flight." She had advised Jeremy to save the battery on his phone that she would use the Internet for news of his flight and that we were aware of what was happening to him.

Later, Jeremy told Donna that within a few minutes after take-off, all the cabin lights had gone off, and they flew the rest of the way with only the emergency lights down the center! Jeremy had already eaten the few snacks he packed from his Easter basket and what he was able to buy at a nearby kiosk because the airline announced that passengers were not to the leave the area. Once he boarded the plane, he thought he would get something to eat — Not so! Why? Because they only take credit cards! Ten hours after Jeremy arrived at the airport, the plane finally landed, and Aunt Donna was there to pick him up at 5:30 a.m.! When I hung up from Donna's call that she had our boy in Niagara Falls, I just broke down and cried (again — where were these tears coming from?) ♀

A nurse came rushing into my room to check my monitor. She saw that I was awake and I told her I would be OK in a few minutes. Then in the dim light, she saw Jerr laying on the leather chair which flattened out to a bed which he had been given to sleep and saw that the sheet had come off him. Our room had always been freezing, and I had two blankets on me. She went to go pull the "sheet" down over his legs, and we heard Jerr say "Wha- wha -what's going on?!" She had mistakenly pulled on his white cargo shorts instead! I whispered to the nurse, "Aha, I know what you were doing to my husband when you thought I was asleep! " We all quietly laughed and laughed with tears in our eyes. And every time she came into my room, she would have a great, big smile on her face. 🔱 🔱

(Later, I wrote Spirit Airlines about Jeremy's experience — and their response? They sent Jeremy a credit voucher for a future flight — OMG!)

The next two days with Jerr spending nights and day with me, I remained in "abnormal sinus rhythm" from an atrial fibrillation condition. The doctor scheduled me in the Cath Lab where he would shock my heart back to normal — hopefully. I waited all day in terror for this to be done, in spite of being told "it's a simple procedure." *(Sure! You say!)* Finally mid-afternoon, I was taken down with Jerr accompanying me. I waited another hour signing paperwork for the procedure. Finally, I was taken into the Cath room, where four or five people were awaiting the doctor and anesthesiologist. I looked up at the ceiling and in a slight fog, I saw Debra's face! I gasped and was going to start crying when a young Indian doctor rushed into the room, looked at the computer and said "Abort, abort, she's now in normal sinus rhythm!"

He left the room to report to my doctor. The team looked at each other and eventually they were dismissed for the day. I lay there alone for several minutes, looked back at the ceiling and was calling "Debra, Debra!" When Jerr was brought back to the lab, I told him what had happened, he leaned down and hugged me, and we were both in tears. I whispered, "I saw Debra!" My doctor came in and tweeked my toe and said "Damn you, damn you!" The three of us always joke with each other. 🔱 🔱 "Dr. B., you are a wonderful doctor." He threw his arms up and said, "I didn't do anything." I said, "That's why you are a wonderful doctor!" He said, "I'll see you upstairs tomorrow morning."

The nurse then came in with a smile and said, "You remember the hour we spent signing paperwork for this procedure? Well, there is just as much paperwork to cancel it as there was to approve it! I'll get all the papers ready and you can go back upstairs. It was 1-½ hours before I returned to my room at 8:30 p.m. — twenty-seven hours since I had last eaten and eventually I was given my dinner. The next day, I was discharged. Much later, I cried. "Debra, Oh, Debra!" Did we now have an angel watching over us? Another one of Debra's gifts?

One and a half months later, Jerr said, "Let's leave, sweetheart." So here I start arrangements for a flight, for the transport of our car and returning to Williamsville.

Jerr and I hosted Debra's Memorial Lunch at the Hickory Hill clubhouse on June 26th for about 50 family and friends. Debra's birthday would have been June 28th. Displayed on a lit candle was Debra's picture, then the three storyboards, a few other photos and the Guestbook given us by the funeral home which guests signed. We did not arrange a memorial ceremony with a priest or prayers because this was yet another "celebration of Debra's life." My heart almost stopped when I saw Dr. Yi from OCC Oncology come into the door! I just went up to him and I hugged him (*Was it appropriate?!*) I introduced him to others as everyone had heard of Debra's wonderful experience with Dr. Yi and OCC Oncology!

During lunch, we had a pleasant discussion with the friends at our table, and then Dr. Yi turned to me and stated, "I never answered the question in your 'thank you' letter about a foundation, but we've now put one in place, and it should be completed within a few weeks! We'll work on it when it's ready!"

(*Hallelujah! So many people had asked me where to make a contribution and because I was unsure, they made them to their favorite charities. All I knew was I didn't want them going to RPCI or the American Cancer Society. Now they can go to the new foundation! Another gift?*)

(*Debra, did you see that Dr. Yi gave us the honor of attending your luncheon? He saw all your photos and signed the Guest Book. So, yes, sweetheart, we did get to meet him, and I know you were in the room with us!)*

5/1/12 —

Petitioned prayers to St. Jude for Debra's soul. (*In spite of my faith, there are so many puzzling and frightening thoughts about death. But suddenly I remember, "The Virgin Mary said, "Do not forsake your faith, for in the end, it will be all that remains."*)

5/13/12, Mother's Day, —

Jeremy's message to his mother on Facebook was:

"Sometimes I think of my mother, and I wonder when you heal.
How and when do you survive, and when does it become real.
The pain of losing loved ones, it hurts so deep inside,

You simply want to run away, escape, or somehow hide.
When mom first got sick, I knew I had to be strong.
I think I really didn't believe; the reports just had to be wrong.

Sometimes she seemed to be better; she seemed to be doing OK.
Then all of sudden, she'd be worse; it changed from day to day.
For 3 years, mom fought stomach cancer, a battle she finally lost,
I didn't want to see her suffer, no matter what the cost.
She lay so quiet, she lay so still,
And I prayed for God to have HIS WILL.
It's been 3 months, since she died that day,

And I know she's in heaven, and she's OK.
I try not to be selfish, but I don't understand,
What was her purpose, and what God's plan was.
I pray for God's blessings, that's all I can say,

And once again to tell you, Mom, Happy Mothers Day.

I love you, Mom, forever and always, Jeremy ♥"

Jeremy, selfishness applies when you don't care who gets hurt as long as you get what you want. That isn't you, you do care!

June 2012 —

We went to Canalfest in Tonawanda and then to the Erie County Fair in Hamburg.

6/29/12, Fri. — Day after Debra's birthday —

Jeremy on Facebook: "Some times I just sit here and wish my mom was here!"

7/1/12 —

We gave a donation to Compassionate Friends so that in their Walk to Remember in memory of Debra, her name/photo would be carried by Walk participants. This year the walk was held on Sunday, 7/22/12 in Costa Mesa, California. An acknowledgement was sent by their member services department in Oak Brook, Illinois.

8/3/12, Fri. —

Donna informed us Debra's headstone was finally in. The grass will grow eventually, she thought the ivy went all the way around the headstone, but it's only in the center and that it was smaller than the example she was shown. We made arrangements to meet at the cemetery. She talked about Debra and how she felt MSMH staff were rushing her out too quickly, the nun was rude, and yet Debra always tried to maintain a positive outlook — in spite of what was done to her and no matter how someone treated her. She was told "Let it go, you're in denial!" She was always fighting for Dilaudid. There are so many pain medications — why? Because some people respond better to one over another. She was so hungry, wanted to eat.

8/25/12 —

Jeremy starts school on Sept. 5, his senior year. He's involved
not only as a DJ in the entire area but in League bowling
and basketball.

9/1/12 —

We go to the Lewiston Peach Festival, then stop at the cemetery
to say a prayer for Debra, remembering the year before when we
brought her a huge peach shortcake and a can of whipped cream!

I still feel Debra's spirit. On one of my down days, I turned the
page on a book I was reading and this message jumps out at me
— *"You ask what is the meaning of this? Why must there always be a
meaning. Can you not accept what the Lord has done without question?"*

It is so painful and every day there are snippets of occasions when
we remember something of Debra's happy spirit or laughter,
things she said, or how we used to sit in the living room with Jerr
and watch Jeopardy. Or we how we now mention a restaurant,
and Jerr would begin to say, "Call D...." I know the pain will
never go away but with all the family and friends and the beautiful
things they did for us and what others wrote and gifted in Debra's
memory, and now this book. And it makes me realize that in
spite of the tears and pain and the loss of my beloved daughter,
how grateful I am, and it reminds me of what Benedictine monk
Brother David Steindl-Rast wrote:

*"You think this is just another day in your life. It's not just another day.
It's the one day that was given to you. Today. It's given to you. It's a gift.
It's the only gift you have right now. And the only appropriate response is
gratefulness.....If you do nothing else, cultivate that response to the great
gift of this unique day. If you learn to respond as if it was the first day
of your life......and as if it would be your last day, then you will spend
this day very well.....as you look at the eyes of people, each one has an
incredible story and that story is in part from their ancestors. Half of*

the people you meet could never fully fathom your story. Open your heart to the incredible gift that civilization gives to us. Wish that you open your heart to all these blessings. Everyone you meet on this day might be impressed by you, by your eyes, your smile, your touch and just by your presence. Let the gratefulness overflow into blessings, then it will be blessed by you — and it will then really be a good day!"

10/26/12 —

Jeremy buys his Mitsubishi car, light orange, and loaded, part from his mother's estate, which we gave him. I also gave him Debra's picture for the sun visor — the one where she has such a joyous smile. The car fulfills yet another wish from his Mom's "Bucket List!"

11/23/12 —

Donna, Jerr and I had an unexpected cruise to celebrate our three birthdays! It started with a casual conversation over breakfast with Terri, and Mark, when she said, " I want to do something. You know, there's a mini-cruise we can take." She and Mark had taken that cruise before and said we'd love it. Jerr turned to me and said, "Call Donna and ask her if she can go." Donna called back in a few hours that not only had she arranged time off work but was able to get a seat on a flight on Thanksgiving Day! (She used the remainder of her Jet Blue voucher credit!) When I made our reservations, we got one of the last three family rooms left. I went to church and then we went to the airport to get our little girl. I made a small but very special Thanksgiving dinner at home, we lit Debra's candle, and we felt she was with us.

"Oh, my God, I humbly ask Your forgiveness for what I said to You. Thank you for the gift of my daughters, Debra and Donna, and for the gift of Jerr and Jeremy, and in your mercy bless us. Thank you for my life, for my family and friends. These are blessed gifts to us!"

11/24/12 - Royal Caribbean Cruise

The three of us departed from Miami on our cruise, meeting up with Terri and Mark on the ship. What a special time together! We needed that. Donna gave us little gifts — a money clip for Jerr and a Royal Caribbean Christmas ornament which I keep on our mirrored shelf in our dining room. We agreed to observe Thanksgiving and our birthdays on the same ship next year, God willing!

Jeremy has found a girlfriend — a lovely young lady — and he seems to be happy again. Her family sounds like very special, loving people. I can hardly wait to meet them.

Donna has found a place to live, a job near home, a new car, and seems to have recovered from the painful medical symptoms. She is a happier person and has spent more time with Jeremy and his girlfriend, getting to know each other. Donna baked Christmas cookies with them and spent some time during Christmas. She plans to go skating or sledding with them. and it's so gratifying that this relationship is now developing oops, never mind.

12/22/12 - Donna's gift

A large fruit box was delivered with Donna's message: Dear Mom & Jerry, It's not a holiday gift, it is just a Thank You for being there Love, Donna, Jim, Jeremy! Fruit, fruit, fruit!

2/23/13 - Jeremy's Facebook:

"Yesterday was a year since my mom has been gone. I miss her truly to death and I would seriously do anything to get her back. She was the best mom anybody could ever had, and she made my life amazing. I will always remember all the memories that I had with her and I promise they will never go away. I love you mom forever and always ♥"

2/24/13 - Debra's first anniversary.

We had a memorial mass at St. Matthew. Jerr, Terry and friends from church attended. For two weeks, I had plan to call and ask if Father Valle could do the Mass even though it was not scheduled that weekend, could the Dora sing my favorite songs, could I order flowers....... and something always interfered. Sunday, I walked in and Father was celebrating the Mass and played his guitar! His homily was about his mentor and friend who had just passed away. Father selected a phrase from the gospel from Luke (Luke 6:28-26), and his final phrase was, "I saw the face of Jesus!"

The Communion anthem was another of my favorite pieces, "Be Not Afraid... I go before you always, come follow me and I will give you peace!" Had Debra just planned her own Mass — another gift to me?! I just sobbed! *(Please, God, let it be so — that she saw the face of Jesus! Thank you, Jesus!)*

2/28/13 - Jeremy's Facebook:

Dear Mom.... You don't even know how much I miss you so far. Every day I'm not in the best mood because I know that you are not by my side. I gave you a lot of promises before you passed away and some of these I achieved and some of these I didn't yet. But don't think I wont because I will always do anything for you. Mom, you were always there for me when I needed you, always making me dinner and supporting me all the way up till know now. I hate to see you go but at least you are not suffering any more and if things work out with the girl I told you about, I promise I will achieve the other goals. I promise to come visit you every time I am out in Niagara Falls whether anybody goes or not. I love you, Mom, so much. Your Son Jeremy ©

.........and so life goes on.......

1 Corinthians 13:13: Faith, hope and love remain, these three; but the greatest of these is love.

# # # #

I'M FREE

Don't grieve for me, for now I'm free.
I'm following the path God has laid, you see.
I took His hand when I heard His call.
I turned my back and left it all.
I could not stay another day.
To laugh, to love, to work or play.
Tasks left undone must stay that way.
I've found the peace at the close of day.
If my parting has left a void,
Then fill it with remembered joys.
A friendship shared, a laugh, a kiss.
Oh yes, these things I too will miss.
Be not burdened with times of sorrow.
I wish you the sunshine of tomorrow.
My life's been full, I favored much,
Good friends, good times, a loved one's touch.
Perhaps my time seemed all too brief.
Don't lengthen it now with undue grief,
Lift up your hearts and peace to thee.
God wanted me now, He set me free.

I AM NOT THERE

Do not stand at my grave and weep,
I am not there, I do not sleep.
I am in a thousand winds that blow,
I am the softly falling snow.
I am the gentle showers of rain,
I am in the fields of ripening grain.
I am in the morning hush,
I am in the graceful rush
Of birds in circling flight.
I am the star shine of the night.
I am in the flowers that bloom,
I am in a quiet room,
I am the birds that sing,
I am in each lovely thing.
Do not stand at my grave and weep.
I am not there.
I did not die!
By Mary Frye

Both poems from Claudia, Lorraine's Mary Kay Consultant.

3/25/12

ACKNOWLEDGEMENTS

First and foremost, to my husband, **Jerr**: The source of strength and love, — the common sense voice in a world filled with the cacophony of confusion and deceit. You are God's gift to me and our family. So, OK, God made a tiny oversight — you're Jewish and I'm Catholic!

To my families:

Debra: Your light, laugher, love and gentleness will be gifts to us always.

Donna: My little peanut dynamo, such a brilliant artist, a creative woman, a multi-tasker! May you find the happiness that I have. Remember when you and Debra used to say "If toucan, we can!" You were always together, she'll be with you always.

Jeremy, our grandson: You are a wonderful young man; you have grown in maturity. You get your artistic talents and quiet demeanor from your Mother but your musical talents from me, and your creativeness from both Donna and me — aren't you lucky! You have found a great talent as a DJ. You work to achieve the goals you have set — never forget this as they will help you in the future. May you always have your Mom in heaven watching over you in everything you do. You were her life, sweetheart, she loved you so much. And you have us on earth to hug you, love you, to be there for you, and watch over you, too! And may you find a lovely young lady to love you as you love her. Your Mom will see to that!

Tia Connie: The embodiment of the "mother" heart that I missed my whole life. Tia, you are a fantastic woman; the keeper of all the memories in our family. You keep all of us together with your phone calls and sometimes your gentle scolding because of the truth, yet the laughter and joy is always present. Thanks for the laughter and the tears — both were healing. To Annie and all the families on the West Coast, your phone calls, cards, offers of help were so special.

Chickie and Steve, Janet, Amy, Stephen and their spouses, sons and daughters: Having you there when we needed it most — putting your personal lives aside at the last minute — meant the world to us.

Erma and Lou: Your emails through the three years, the special gifts and contributions in Debra's name, all the smiles and the tears, the encouraging words and the insightful truth we shared as we now have a common bond — the passing of our children.

Frankie and Sarah: Thanks for thinking of us, for your love, and your calls and contributions.

Mark and Sally: With gratitude for all you shared over the years, never forgetting our daughters and especially Debra in her last years. Your prayers, your notes and cards, your calls, your contributions, your thoughtfulness, and your presence — even in spite of your own health challenges — was so comforting to us.

Midge and Bill and family: You have no idea how blessed your visit to Debra was and your blessing her in her last hours. In spite of your own challenges with cancer, you ministered to her. God bless you for that.

Connie and Nick: Your "memory" emails were so special and your message in the Guest Book was so telling of your memory of Debra. You later told me you remembered her wonderful personality and her infectious zest for life and how hard it's been for Donna as she lost her "partner in crime!"

Brenda and Robin of England: Best friends for fifty-five years and who extended the most gracious hospitality. Your astonishing surprise trip through England, France, Austria and Germany where we shared the awesome, spiritual experience of Oberammergau (produced once every ten years)! Then later our trips throughout the British Isles, Scotland, Ireland, and Wales — memories that will be with me always. Sharing Rotary with Robin and his colleagues was always special, receiving the gracious welcome at meetings during a time when women were not involved in Rotary in England! To the rest of my friends in England, you will always be so special to me for your hospitality, your letters and cards through the years — and even today through emails.

To our extended family and our best friends: We embrace you, we love you all, and you each know why —

Terri and Mark, Bill and Jo-Ann and Debbie and Hunter, Sue and Fred, Gloria and Mike, Sereda, Renee, Mario and Gina, and the rest of the Library group and in memoriam — Linda, Edie, Mildred (who each shared this walk with me) — all the rest of our wonderful friends at The Hallmark, space does not allow me to list your names.

Sandra and Lew and all the friends at Hickory Hill Estates and each and every person who attended Debra's Memorial lunch, your cards and gifts. You are special friends.

Alan and Shelly and friends of the local political party in Hollywood and what you, your tears and hugs meant to me. Thank you, too, for being there and for your touching tribute to Debra at one of the meetings.

Bea and Bob and the lasting friendships of Rotary International and other Rotarian friends throughout the years, both here in the

United States and in England. In an organization that has members believing in the same values, principles, and goals, you develop close ties for all times.

Friends in Washington, DC throughout all these years — professional people who opened a whole new world, who trusted my instincts in our projects, and became lifelong friends — Ambassador John M., Harold O. and the kindness of Mrs. Virginia K. of the White House.......

Friends from the (then) NYS Seaway Trail — An seemingly impossible task when Assemblyman M. called 19 of us together, but with hard work, plans, fun, and the loss of dear people, we still remain friends, and leave a legacy to be enjoyed by thousands.

Dr. Yi, Dr. Yap and every member of the staff at OCC Oncology: Please know how special you were to Debra and to our family in her final months — I repeat, she said you gave her back her womanhood and humanity. That was the greatest gift!

May you all be blessed! With all our love!

# # # #

REFERENCES

Cancercare.com for informational literature. "Helping teenagers cope with death of a parent."

Cancer Treatment Centers of America (CTCA), www.cancercenters.com

Chimayo Mission, Santa Fe, New Mexico

Millard Fillmore Suburban Hospital, Williamsville, NY

Mount Saint Mary's Hospital, Lewiston, New York

New River Gorge Bridge, West Virginia

Niagara Falls Memorial Medical Hospital, Niagara Falls, New York

OCC Oncology, Williamsville, NY

Oberammagau, "The Passion Play", Germany

Roswell Park Cancer Institute, www.roswellpark.org

St. Jude Children's Research Hospital, www.*stjude.org*

St. Jude Shrine, 512 S. Saratoga Street, Baltimore, MD 21201 (410) 685-3063.

Tamarack, Beckley, West Virginia

Google: www.thebible.com, clic on Bible Search.

The Compassionate Friends — www.compassionatefriends.org.
Supporting family after a child dies.

INDEX

Our medical research was necessitated by our naiveté in this process. Tests and unpronounceable medications were tossed at us. Information is available to anyone through the Internet, although the majority of my research was through WebMD. Refer to it further for videos, audio, warnings, uses, side effects, precautions, interactions, or overdoses.

* www.WEBMD — *Better Information-Better Health*

©2005-2013 WebMD, LLC. All rights reserved.

Johns Hopkins Cancer Update, May 5, 2010, includes what cancer cells feed on.

CPSIA information can be obtained at www.ICGtesting.com
Printed in the USA
BVOW07s1133120813

328218BV00001B/34/P